Atlas of General Thoracic Surgery

Atlas of General Thoracic Surgery

Larry R. Kaiser, M.D.
Professor of Surgery
The University of Pennsylvania
Director, General Thoracic Surgery
Hospital of The University of Pennsylvania
Philadelphia, Pennsylvania

Tracie A. Aretz, M.S.M.I.
Medical Illustrator
Glenside, Pennsylvania

with 251 *illustrations*

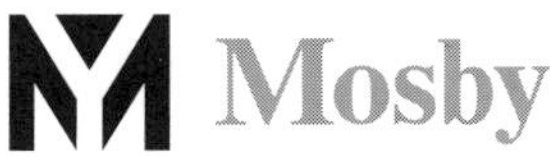

St. Louis Baltimore Boston Carlsbad Chicago Naples New York Philadelphia Portland
London Madrid Mexico City Singapore Sydney Tokyo Toronto Wiesbaden

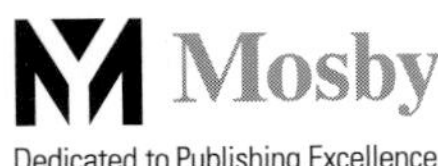

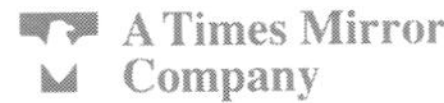

Vice President and Publisher: Anne S. Patterson
Editor: Michael Brown
Developmental Editor: Becca Gruliow
Editorial Assistant: Marla Sussman
Project Manager: Linda Clarke
Senior Production Editor: Allan S. Kleinberg
Composition Specialists: Steven Cavanaugh, Pamela Merritt, and Christine Boles
Designer: Carolyn O'Brien
Manufacturing Manager: Bill Winneberger

Printed in the United States of America
Composition by Mosby Electronic Production, Philadelphia
Printing/binding by Maple Vail Book Manufacturing Group–York

Mosby–Year Book, Inc.
11830 Westline Industrial Drive
St. Louis, Missouri 63146

Library of Congress Cataloging-in-Publication Data
Kaiser, Larry R.
Atlas of general thoracic surgery / by Larry R. Kaiser
p. cm.
Includes bibliographical references and index.
ISBN 0-8016-6380-6
1. Chest—Surgery—Atlases. I. Title.
[DNLM: 1. Lung Diseases—surgery—atlases. 2. Thoracic Surgery—methods—atlases. 3. Esophageal Diseases—surgery—atlases. WF 17K13a 1997]
RD536.K37 1997
617.5′4059—dc20
DNLM/DLC
for Library of Congress 96-29148
CIP

97 98 99 00 01 / 9 8 7 6 5 4 3 2 1

This book is dedicated to the memory of two men whose lives and wisdom continue to guide me. First to my dad, Jerry Kaiser, who died much too young and with whom I never had the opportunity to share the joys of my adult personal or professional life. I think he would have been proud. And to Nate Burns, patient, friend, and wise counselor, who in so many ways reminded me of my father.

To Ruthy, Jonathan, and Jeffrey for their never-ending love and support.

PREFACE

In this book I have attempted to cover the specialty of general thoracic surgery from such rudimentary procedures as chest tube insertion to the complex nuances of lung transplantation. I have attempted to provide more than an atlas. Tracie Aretz, a superb medical illustrator, came into the operating room and has faithfully and magnificently depicted the surgical procedures. But the book is more than illustrations with captions. It is a *practice* of thoracic surgery distilled from the training I was fortunate to receive from the leading individuals in the field and from eleven years of teaching general and thoracic surgery residents.

Of course, there are many ways to perform a given operative procedure; there is no one right way. I have tried to demonstrate techniques that have stood the test of time and that have proven safe, reliable, and expeditious. Where applicable, I have detailed potential problem areas and how to avoid them. Trouble in thoracic surgery is far better avoided, no matter how talented one is at fixing the problem. Avoiding problems requires a thorough working knowledge of the anatomy and experience in performing the operation. This book is intended to serve both as a guide for the trainee new to thoracic surgery and as a review source for the experienced surgeon who may perform some of these procedures only ocassionally. I have attempted to be comprehensive in the scope of the procedures covered and in so doing to provide a solid foundation for extending this knowledge to more complex, unique problems, which may arise in the care of patients with thoracic pathology.

I am indebted to Joel Cooper, first and always mentor but later partner at Washington University in St. Louis, Griff Pearson, Bob Ginsberg, Tom Todd, Alec Patterson, and Clem Hiebert, all at the University of Toronto at the time of my residency. I am also grateful to Nael Martini and Manjit Bains, colleagues at Memorial Sloan-Kettering Cancer Center, my first post-residency position, who not only tolerated me but encouraged and nurtured me as a young attending surgeon.

Larry R. Kaiser

INTRODUCTION

The specialty of Thoracic Surgery arose from the ranks of General Surgery when it became clear that surgical problems of the chest demanded, if not special expertise, at least special interest. The specialty initially was devoted to the care of patients with complications caused mainly by the ravages of tuberculosis. A major impetus to the development of the specialty was provided by the publication of Graham's classic monograph, "Empyema Thoracis", which arose from the work of the Empyema Commission. The recognition of the principles involved in treating empyema resulted in a seven-fold reduction in mortality from this complication of hemolytic streptococcus infections of the respiratory tract at a time that predated antibiotic therapy.

The era of cardiac surgery marked a major shift in the direction of the specialty of Thoracic Surgery and an entirely new breed of surgeon. Diseases of the chest not involving the heart took a subordinate position in all but a few training programs in this country. Certainly pulmonary surgery was being done by thoracic surgeons but almost always in a secondary position. Perhaps owing to the development of lung transplantation, thoracic surgery, as a distinct component of the specialty of Cardiothoracic Surgery, is back. Heart surgery, of course, is still going strong, but no longer is the "non-cardiac" specialist taking a back seat. Essentially every training program has at least one individual who specializes in general thoracic surgery, and a few programs even have a separate track for the training of such individuals. The general thoracic surgeon needs to have a solid background and in-depth knowledge of oncology, pulmonary medicine, gastroenterology, and surgical pathology. The education of the general thoracic surgeon is every bit as specialized as that of the cardiac surgeon, perhaps more so. Hopefully this book will contribute to the education and training of all cardiothoracic surgeons, whether they intend to make general thoracic surgery their life's work or just an occasional diversion from cardiac surgery. The book should also be of benefit to the education of general surgery residents who rotate through the thoracic surgical service and to those general surgeons who as part of their practice perform thoracic surgical procedures.

Larry R. Kaiser

CONTENTS

PART I

Diagnostic Procedures

PART II

Therapeutic Procedures

PART III

Thoracic Incisions

PART IV

Pulmonary Resections

PART V

Chest Wall Procedures

PART VI

Miscellaneous Procedures

PART VII

Lung Transplantation

PART VIII

Tracheal Resection

PART IX

The Esophagus

PART I

Diagnostic Procedures

CHAPTER 1

Rigid Bronchoscopy

With the advent of the flexible fiberoptic bronchoscope, rigid bronchoscopy is in danger of becoming a lost art. Though used less, rigid bronchoscopy remains an important tool to the thoracic surgeon mainly for therapeutic purposes. It is essential that trainees from thoracic surgical programs be competent in performing rigid bronchoscopy, since the procedure can be lifesaving. Indications for rigid bronchoscopy include the management of massive hemoptysis, removal of foreign bodies, debulking of lesions obstructing the airway, emergency establishment of an airway, assessment of airway invasion by esophageal carcinoma, use of the laser, stent placement, and assessment of tracheal lesions in preparation for resection.

DESCRIPTION OF THE PROCEDURE

The technique is relatively simple, but it takes a considerable amount of practice to get the feel of it. The patient is positioned supine with the head supported in a "sniffing" position (**Fig. 1-1**); that is, the neck should be slightly flexed, not hyperextended, when the instrument is introduced. The instrument is introduced with the bevel down and the tip of the epiglottis visualized (**Fig. 1-2**). This is the key move in this procedure: the epiglottis must be seen. Once the epiglottis is seen, the tip of the bronchoscope is used to lift the epiglottis to visualize the vocal cords. The instrument is brought underneath the epiglottis but only slightly so, since going too far inferiorly places the instrument behind the larynx. Slipping the instrument just beneath the epiglottis and lifting, with the operator using his or her thumb and not the patient's teeth as a fulcrum, allows the vocal cords to be well seen. The bronchoscope is rotated 90 degrees, slid past the vocal cords, and then rotated back to its original position (**Fig. 1-3**). The pillow supporting the head is removed once the instrument has been introduced so that the neck is slightly extended.

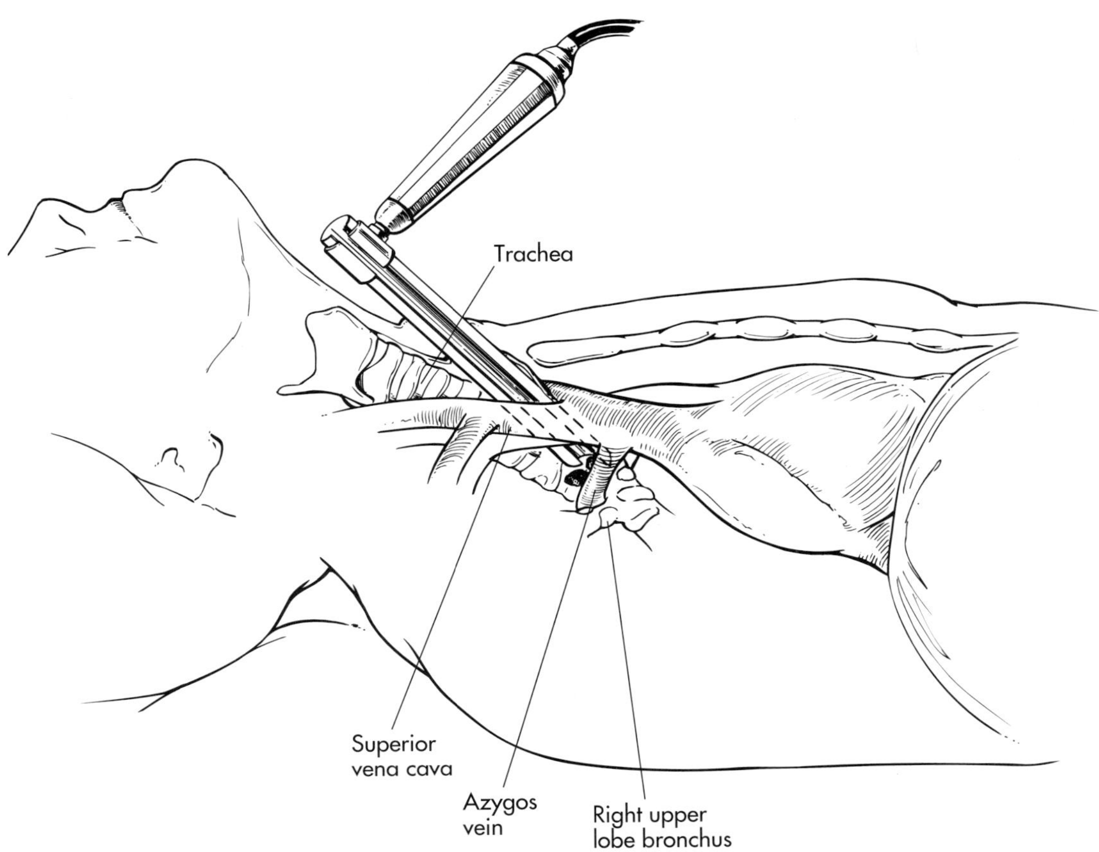

FIGURE 2-2

tors) are inserted and pulled laterally and superiorly to retract the thyroid gland superiorly. The pretracheal fascia is incised, a key move, and swept off the trachea with a sweeping motion of the closed scissors. I insert a finger into the mediastinal plane just anterior to the trachea and bluntly dissect the mediastinal plane. The innominate artery is felt coursing anteriorly across the finger, and the aortic arch is also noted. The right and left paratracheal areas are palpated. In many patients the carina may be palpated, but it is rarely possible to palpate the subcarinal space. The carina is evident by palpating not just the right and left main bronchi but by palpating the softer area of the anterior trachea at the carina. If lymph nodes are palpable, usually along the right paratracheal area, the finger is used to dissect this area to facilitate dissection through the scope.

When the dissection is performed correctly, the mediastinoscope is easy to insert (**Fig. 2-1, *inset***). A variety of mediastinoscopes are available, and the surgeon needs to become comfortable with the instrument chosen. If the instrument is difficult to insert, slightly rotating it usually allows it to be placed (**Fig. 2-2**). If no pathology is palpable, I begin the dissection in the right tracheobronchial area (level 4) since this location is richest in lymph nodes. Dissection is performed with the suction, and countertraction is obtained by impinging the structures to be dissected with the end of the mediastinoscope. Once a lymph node is visualized and "palpated" with the suction tip, a biopsy is taken. A needle may be used to aspirate a structure prior to biopsy and, even if blood is not seen in the syringe, the structure should be observed for bleeding after the needle is withdrawn. No attempt is made to remove the entire lymph node, and I use a twisting motion, not a direct pull, to remove the piece. Pieces of lymph node come easily; other structures do not. I use a blunt, noncutting type of biopsy forceps usually used for laryngeal biopsies and never pull with much force. If the piece grasped does not come easily, I stop and reassess, perhaps even doing further dissection with the suction tip. Biopsies are taken of other nodal locations, specifically the right level 2 area (paratracheal), the level 7 area (subcarinal), and the left level 4 location (tracheobronchial angle).

If there is a palpable lymph node or mass, a biopsy of this structure is done first and may be all that is required. A cardinal rule I follow when performing mediastinoscopy is to avoid greed. I take what I need and get out. Once I have documented unilateral disease it is important to exclude the presence of contralateral disease (N3); I therefore sample nodes from the opposite side. The surgeon must always know, anatomically, where he is using the trachea as the reference point. Needless to say, the anatomy of the superior mediastinum must be mastered and the surgeon should be well aware of what danger lurks nearby. Structures that can be injured include the innominate artery, azygos vein, right main pulmonary artery, superior vena cava, and left recurrent laryngeal nerve. The most common cause of bleeding during mediastinoscopy is the bronchial arteries in the subcarinal space. This type of bleeding is managed by pressing the mediastinoscope against the bleeding area and using electrocautery, a safe technique as long as the surgeon knows what structures are nearby. Using electrocautery in the vicinity of a major vessel may in itself cause problems. I rarely use electrocautery in the left paratracheal region to avoid injuring the left recurrent laryngeal nerve.

If major bleeding is encountered, the mediastinum should be packed with gauze packing (vaginal packing) as the initial maneuver. Usually the first indication of a major bleed is disappearance of the view through the mediastinoscope into darkness. Because the mediastinum is a small confined space, the bleeding should be controllable with effective packing, providing enough time to perform an appropriate open procedure to manage the hemorrhage. The operative approach to control the bleeding depends somewhat on the structure that is bleeding, thus the importance of knowing where one is anatomically at any given time. By far, the best way of managing catastrophic hemorrhage is to avoid it. If it occurs, median sternotomy should allow access to control the bleeding.

Barring unforeseen complications, once the appropriate biopsies have been obtained hemostasis is checked and the wound closed in two layers. The platysma is reapproximated and the skin closed with a subcuticular suture. If thoracotomy is to follow mediastinoscopy, the specimens are sent for frozen-section analysis; if no tumor is seen, the open procedure follows.

Bibliography

Coughlin M, DesLauriers J, Beaulieu M, et al: Role of mediastinoscopy in pretreatment staging of patients with primary lung cancer, *Ann Thorac Surg* 40:556–560, 1985.

Ginsberg RJ: Evaluation of the mediastinum by invasive techniques, *Surg Clin North Am* 67:1025–1035, 1987.

Patterson GA, Ginsberg RJ, Poon PY, et al: A prospective evaluation of magnetic resonance imaging, computed tomography, and mediastinoscopy in the preoperative assessment of mediastinal node status in bronchogenic carcinoma, *J Thorac Cardiovasc Surg* 94:679–684, 1987.

Pearson FG, Nelems JM, Henderson RD, et al: The role of mediastinoscopy in the selection of treatment for bronchial carcinoma with involvement of superior mediastinal lymph nodes, *J Thorac Cardiovasc Surg* 64:382–390, 1972.

CHAPTER 3

Anterior Mediastinotomy (Chamberlain Procedure)

Anterior mediastinotomy provides additional information about staging that is not obtainable with cervical mediastinoscopy. Tumors of the left upper lobe most commonly metastasize to lymph nodes in the aortopulmonary window, level 5, a location that cannot be accessed by mediastinoscopy. This nodal location is considered mediastinal (N2), but isolated nodal involvement at this location when completely resected carries a significantly better prognosis than any other mediastinal lymph node involvement (approximately 45% after 5 years). Therefore it is reasonable to ask why it is important to initially document nodal disease at this location if the superior mediastinum is negative for tumor as documented by mediastinoscopy. First, the issue of resectability is a critical one and nodal involvement of the aortopulmonary window sometimes renders a tumor unresectable. This is most obvious when the patient presents with left vocal cord paralysis secondary to either the primary tumor or lymph node involvement of the aortopulmonary window with impingement on the left recurrent laryngeal nerve, a situation considered by most to be unresectable. The presence of enlarged lymph nodes in this location as seen on chest CT scan does not deter many surgeons from proceeding immediately to thoracotomy after a negative mediastinoscopy. The lesions in some of these patients will be unresectable. In the interest of entering patients into experimental protocols of neoadjuvant therapy for mediastinal lymph node disease, other surgeons perform either anterior mediastinotomy or videothoracoscopy to document aortopulmonary window nodal involvement.

In addition to providing staging information for tumors of the left upper lobe, anterior mediastinotomy proves useful for the biopsy of a diffuse mediastinal mass where there is a component in the anterior mediastinum. Most commonly, these are lymphomas, but other lesions, such as thymomas or germ cell tumors, occur in this location. For biopsy of a large mediastinal mass, anterior mediastinotomy is a far simpler and quicker procedure than videothoracoscopy. The patient remains supine, a double-lumen endotracheal tube and one-lung ventilation are not required, and larger pieces of material are easier to obtain. The procedure may be performed on either the right or left side.

DESCRIPTION OF THE PROCEDURE

For left anterior mediastinotomy a transverse skin incision is made over the second costal cartilage, found by identifying the cartilage just inferior to the sternal angle (**Fig. 3-1, *inset***). The perichondrium is incised and the second costal cartilage is removed in a subperichondrial plane (**Fig. 3-1**). The

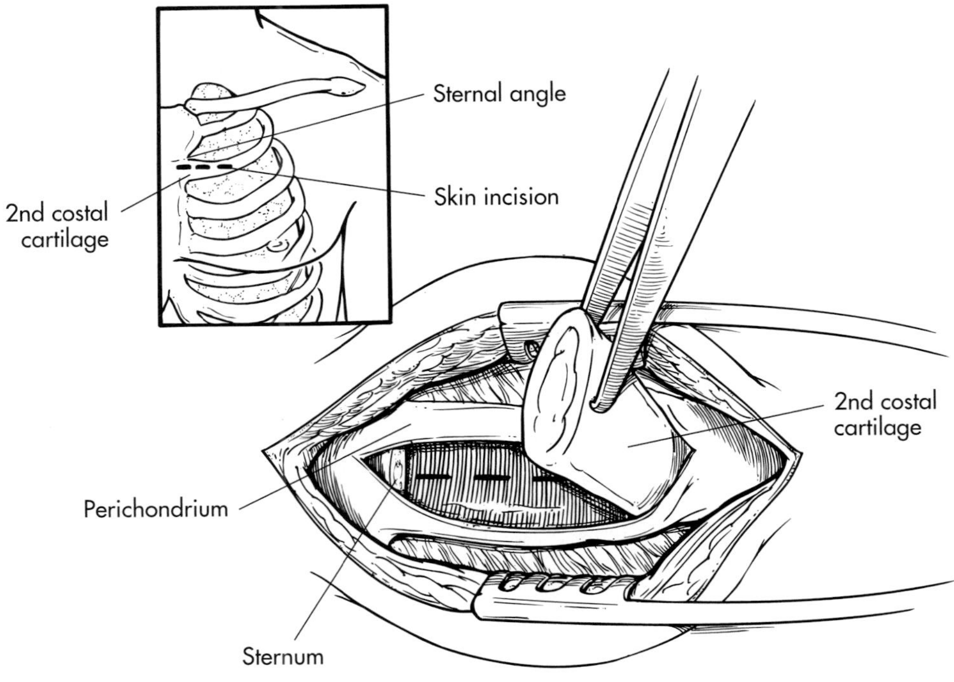

FIGURE 3-1

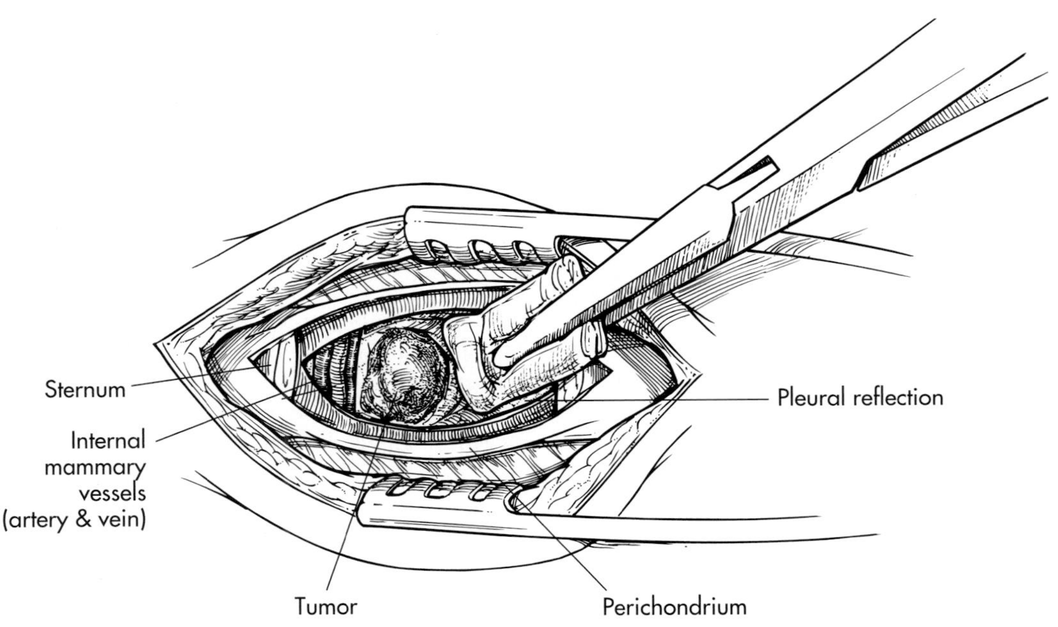

FIGURE 3-2

posterior perichondrium is incised, and care is taken to remain extrapleural within the mediastinum. The pleura is bluntly swept laterally, and the mass comes into view (**Fig. 3-2**). The internal mammary vessels are identified, and if in the way, they are ligated and divided. The mass is palpated, and biopsies are taken either by incising directly into the mass or by using a biopsy forceps. It is important to confirm with frozen-section analysis that diagnostic material has been obtained; thus close cooperation with the pathologist is mandatory. We do not expect necessarily that a definitive diagnosis will be rendered on the basis of frozen section, only an assurance that enough material of good quality has been obtained to permit a diagnosis.

If the pleura is entered inadvertently, a small rubber catheter is placed into the rent and the wound closed in layers. The lung is inflated by the anesthesiologist, and the rubber catheter is removed. At closure no attempt is made to reapproximate the intercostal space, but the posterior perichondrium is sutured. The removal of the second costal cartilage leaves a small residual but noticeable indentation that may be somewhat distressing for the occasional patient; the patient should be forewarned as part of the informed consent.

Bibliography

Ginsberg RJ: Evaluation of the mediastinum by invasive techniques, *Surg Clin North Am* 67:1025–1035, 1987.

McNeill TM and Chamberlain JM: Diagnostic anterior mediastinotomy, *Ann Thorac Surg* 2:532, 1966.

Patterson GA, Piazza D, Pearson FG, et al: Significance of metastatic disease in subaortic lymph nodes, *Ann Thorac Surg* 43:155–159, 1987.

CHAPTER 4

Limited Thoracotomy for Open Lung Biopsy

In patients with a diffuse lung infiltrate where the diagnosis remains unknown, it is often necessary to obtain a piece of lung to provide diagnostic material. Videothoracoscopic techniques recently have been used to obtain pieces of lung tissue but usually require placement of a double-lumen endobronchial tube to effect one-lung ventilation. Occasionally, patients with diffuse lung pathology are critically ill, requiring mechanical ventilation with high inspiratory pressures and FIO_2 just to maintain satisfactory oxygen saturation. To attempt to change the endotracheal tube and replace it with a double-lumen tube carries significant morbidity, not to mention the difficulty in trying to maintain the oxygen saturation while trying to ventilate one lung of the patient. Videothoracoscopy is contraindicated in these patients, and the far easier procedure is a limited anterior thoracotomy.

DESCRIPTION OF THE PROCEDURE

A small inframammary incision is made and carried down onto the chest wall (**Fig. 4-1,** ***inset***). The fourth intercostal space is entered and the lung delivered up into the wound with the aid of a Duval lung clamp (**Fig. 4-1**). Placement of a small rib spreader facilitates exposure. One is limited to taking a biopsy from the portion of lung that is accessible through the small incision. On the left, the lingula and lower lobe are easily found; on the right, the lower lobe usually is sampled. Videothoracoscopy provides the advantage of allowing material from any area of the lung to be sampled. The inframammary incision is aligned usually over the fifth intercostal space, so an effort must be made to make the intercostal opening one space higher. The diaphragm interferes with access to the chest if the fifth space is opened so far anteriorly. The endoscopic linear stapler may be used to remove a piece of lung tissue if the lung cannot be delivered up into the wound.

A chest tube is placed through a separate stab wound, and the wound is closed by reapproximating the pectoralis muscle and the subcutaneous tissue. No attempt is made to place paracostal sutures since the anterior ribs will move very little toward each other. Before the procedure is concluded, material should be submitted for frozen-section analysis to assure that diagnostic material has been

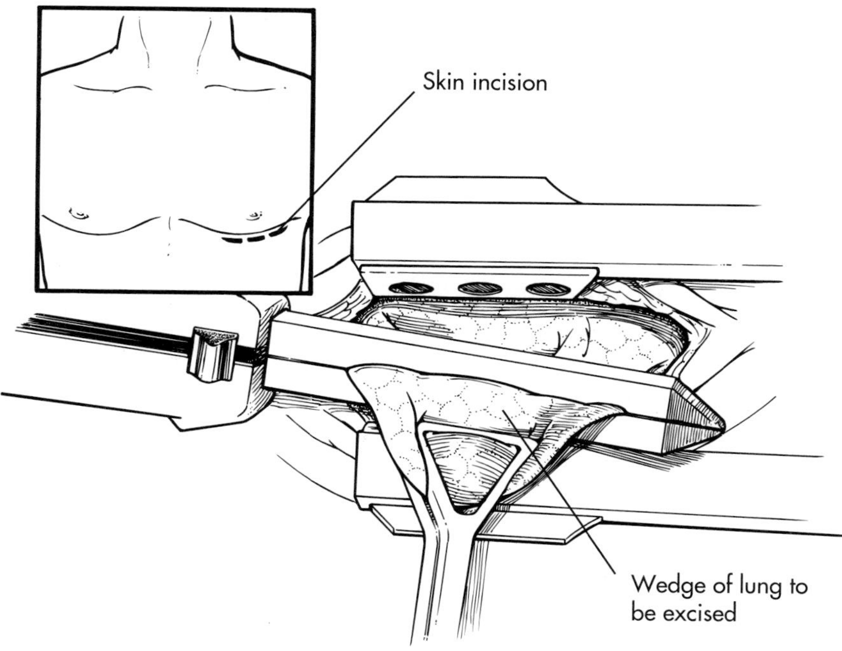

FIGURE 4-1

obtained. If only normal lung has been obtained, further sampling is mandatory. We do not expect the pathologist to render a diagnosis based on the frozen-section result, only to assure us that enough material has been obtained to allow a diagnosis to be made.

Bibliography

Carnochan FM, Walker WS, and Cameron EW: Efficacy of video assisted thoracoscopic lung biopsy: an historical comparison with open lung biopsy, *Thorax* 49:361–363, 1994.

Ferson PF, Landreneau RJ, Dowling RD, et al: Comparison of open versus thoracoscopic lung biopsy for diffuse infiltrative pulmonary disease, *J Thorac Cardiovasc Surg* 106:194–199, 1993.

Gaensler EA and Carrington CB: Open biopsy for chronic diffuse infiltrative lung disease: clinical, roentgenographic and physiological correlations in 502 patients, *Ann Thorac Surg* 30:411–418, 1980.

PART II

Therapeutic Procedures

CHAPTER 5

Tube Thoracostomy

Insertion of a chest tube is a procedure that should be second nature to all surgical residents since it may often be lifesaving. Unfortunately, it is usually assumed that trainees "know" how to insert a chest tube, and frequently no formal instruction is given. Placing a chest tube in the correct location and in a relatively pain-free fashion requires knowledge of certain techniques and experience gained by doing the procedure repeatedly, initially with correct supervision. Most commonly, the ideally located tube passes posteriorly and then up to the apex since the patient spends most of the time supine. For certain indications it may be beneficial to pass the tube inferiorly along the diaphragm. Before insertion of a tube, the chest radiograph should be reviewed and be readily available at the time of insertion. Chest tubes are inserted for drainage of either air or fluid, and the indication for tube insertion determines the size of the tube. For a pneumothorax a smaller tube (22-26 Fr) may be used compared to that used to drain a malignant effusion (28 Fr). To drain blood or pus a larger bore tube should be employed (36–40 Fr).

DESCRIPTION OF THE PROCEDURE

The patient is placed in the supine position with the ipsilateral hand resting behind the head (**Fig. 5-1**). This position results in more accurate tube placement than does the lateral decubitus position. With the patient lying on the side, there is a tendency to insert the tube in a site located too far posteriorly, which is uncomfortable when the patient lies in bed. The tube is inserted through an incision aligned with the anterosuperior iliac spine in approximately the 7th intercostal space. The skin is infiltrated with local anesthetic (1% xylocaine) to raise a wheal. The needle is then directed medially toward the rib and the periosteum is infiltrated. I put the needle directly on the bone to confirm location, then step the needle down to the pleura. The pleura above the rib is infiltrated with local anesthetic. I also perform an intercostal block at least one level above and one level below the proposed tube insertion site. Intravenous sedation may be employed, but a well-placed local anesthetic should prevent significant discomfort for the patient during tube insertion.

Before placing a tube for fluid it is important to demonstrate free-flowing fluid by inserting a needle into the chest. I do not attempt to place a tube unless I get fluid with needle aspiration. Certain effusions are loculated, meaning the lung is adherent in certain locations, and the exact site of the fluid must be located for safe tube insertion. Once I demonstrate free-flowing fluid, a skin incision is made and the scalpel is used to deepen the incision to the intercostal muscle. At the intercostal muscle a hemostat is used to spread the muscle and open it to the level of the pleura (**Fig. 5-2**). The pleu-

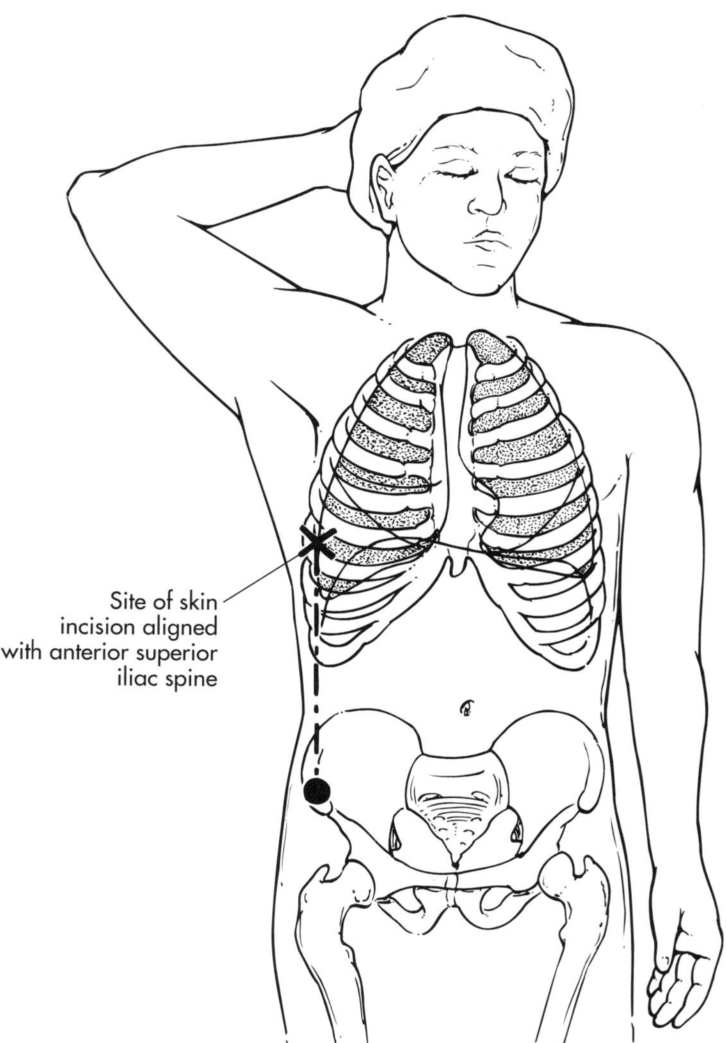

FIGURE 5-1

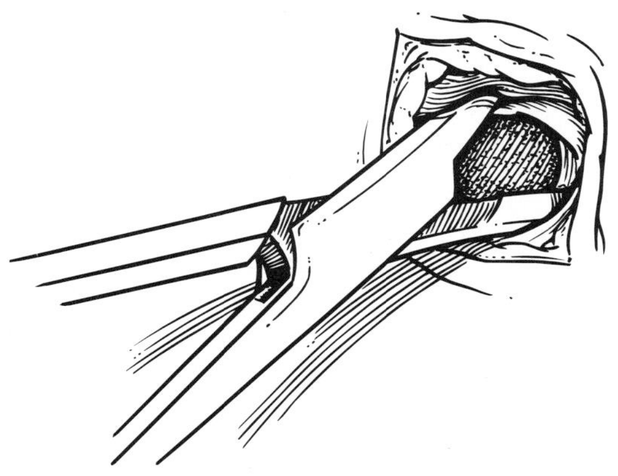

FIGURE 5-2

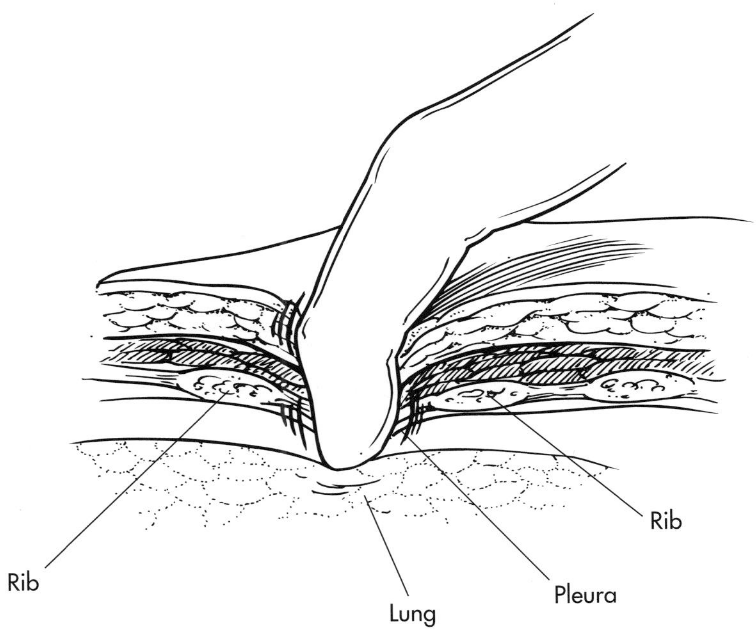

FIGURE 5-3

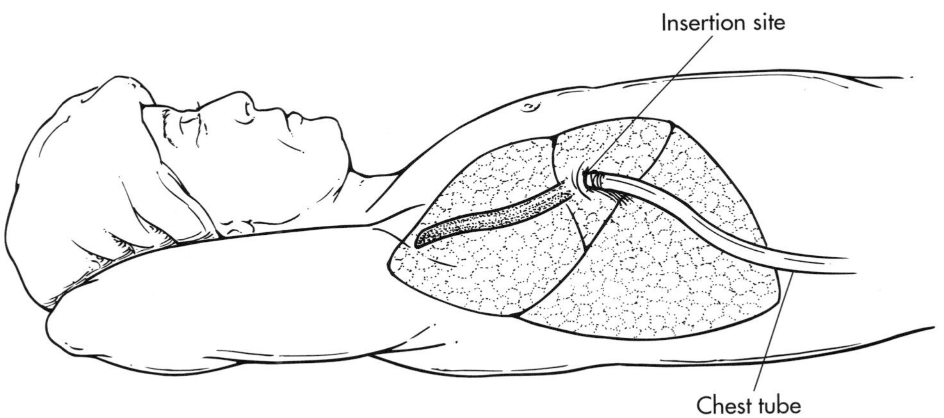

FIGURE 5-4

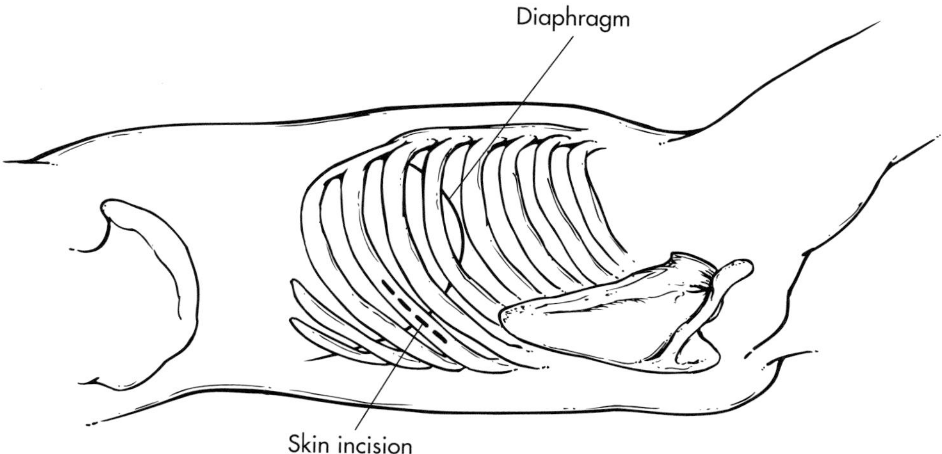

FIGURE 7-1

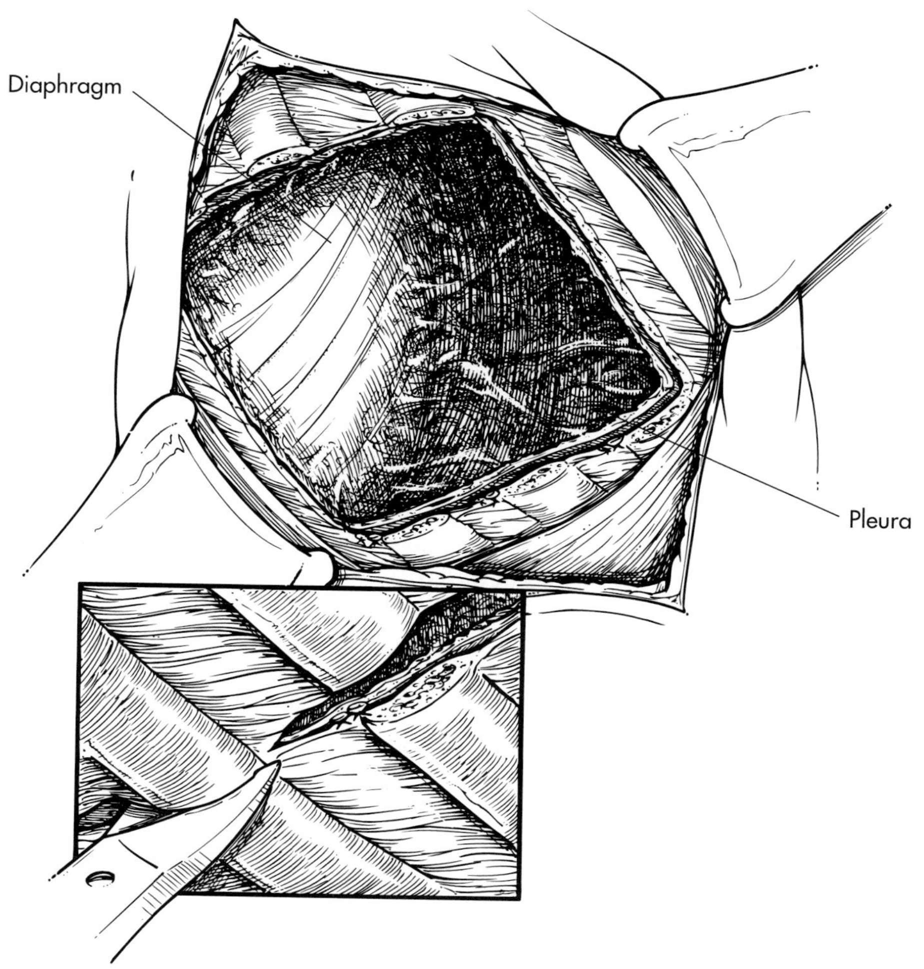

FIGURE 7-2

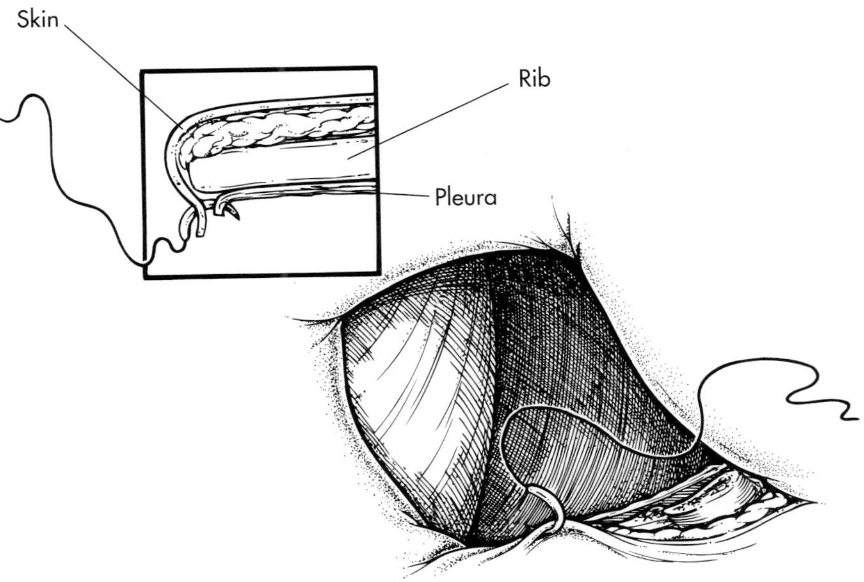

FIGURE 7-3

The space is suctioned and mechanically débrided. If there is an obvious bronchial stump leak, the use of irrigation must proceed with caution. No attempt is made to identify the stump leak, and certainly no attempt is made to repair any leak. The air leak is not the problem; the infected space is the problem and adequate drainage is the solution. Taking two or three ribs usually creates a large enough window to provide excellent drainage. If the scapular tip obscures the window it should be excised, since this obstruction of the window often results in the premature closure of the window. The open window thoracostomy is completed by suturing the skin edges to the edge of thickened pleura with interrupted sutures placed from dermis to pleura so that the skin edge turns in toward the opening (**Fig. 7-3**). The skin edge is brought down to the pleura around the entire circumference of the window. For the first 12 to 14 hours, the window is left loosely packed with saline-moistened gauze. A member of the surgical team should change the first dressing to assess the window. Continued long-term packing of the open window thoracostomy is not necessary. It may even hinder drainage and therefore is discouraged.

Long-term management of open window thoracostomy varies according to the clinical course of the patient. Ultimately, some windows may be closed by transposing a muscle flap into the residual space; others may be closed with the second stage of the classic Clagett procedure, which involves filling the space with antibiotic solution, mobilizing the skin flaps, and suturing the window closed. Many of these windows never come to closure because the patients refuse treatment, not wanting to bother with it, or the windows have spontaneously closed to a size that is not burdensome to the patient.

Currently, filling the space with a flap of transposed muscle is the preferred procedure for management of a chronic space problem and may actually be used in some patients to avoid construction of an open window thoracostomy altogether, though it is a considerably more extensive and complex operation than open window thoracostomy. Often, the condition of the patient who presents with an infected postpneumonectomy space dictates the performance of the less complex procedure at least as the initial management approach.

Bibliography

Cicero R, del Vecchyo C, Porter JK, et al: Open window thoracostomy and plastic surgery with muscle flaps in the treatment of chronic empyema, *Chest* 89:374–377, 1986.

Smolle-Juttner F, Beuster W, Pinter H, et al: Open-window thoracostomy in pleural empyema, *Eur J Cardiothorac Surg* 6:635–638, 1992.

C H A P T E R 8

Videothoracoscopy: General Techniques

A number of books dealing with videothoracoscopy are available, and our purpose here is to delineate general techniques that are applicable to most procedures where these techniques may be used. Indications for videothoracosopy are many and varied, and it is beyond our scope to detail all of them. It is safe to say that videothoracoscopic techniques have become well established in thoracic surgery, and many procedures that formerly required an open thoracotomy may now be performed with this less invasive approach. No compromises are made in the actual operation performed; only access to the chest differs. Technical advances leading to miniaturization of video cameras and refinements in chip technology as well as the development of instruments capable of being used through small incisions have allowed videothoracoscopic techniques to be applied to increasingly complex procedures.

The developments in videothoracoscopy followed the lead of laparoscopy when it was recognized that laparoscopic cholecystectomy was not only feasible but preferable to the open procedure. As opposed to the peritoneal cavity where the working space must be created by insufflation of carbon dioxide gas, the thoracic cavity, with its bony support structure, provides the working space once the lung is collapsed. One-lung ventilation is a standard technique in chest surgery, and without the requirement to maintain a closed environment, as is necessary if gas is to be insufflated, it was quickly realized that small incisions could be made through which instruments could be directly inserted without the need for specialized trocars. Techniques vary considerably among surgeons. The methods presented here work for us because of their simplicity and the rapidity with which the procedures can be accomplished. Many of the techniques fall under the category of video-assisted thoracic surgery, a hybrid between the standard open procedure and a purely endoscopic technique. In this approach, standard instruments inserted through one or more small incisions are used to carry out procedures where most of the visual guidance is provided by the thoracoscope coupled to a miniature video camera. The projection of the image on a video monitor allows the surgeon to work with an assistant on complex procedures.

DESCRIPTION OF THE PROCEDURE

We have developed a series of techniques that essentially standardize the videothoracoscopic approach but allow enough variation to accommodate specialized procedures as necessary. A left endobronchial double-lumen tube is placed to accomplish one-lung ventilation. For almost all procedures, the patient is placed in the lateral decubitus position, as for standard thoracotomy (**Fig. 8-1**). To approach a lesion in the anterior mediastinum, we position the patient with the operated side 30 to 45 degrees from the horizontal, not in full lateral position. The initial incision is made to accommodate the thoracoscope, and I put this incision in the same location for every case. Aligned with the anterior superior iliac spine and in approximately the 7th or 8th intercostal space, a 1-cm

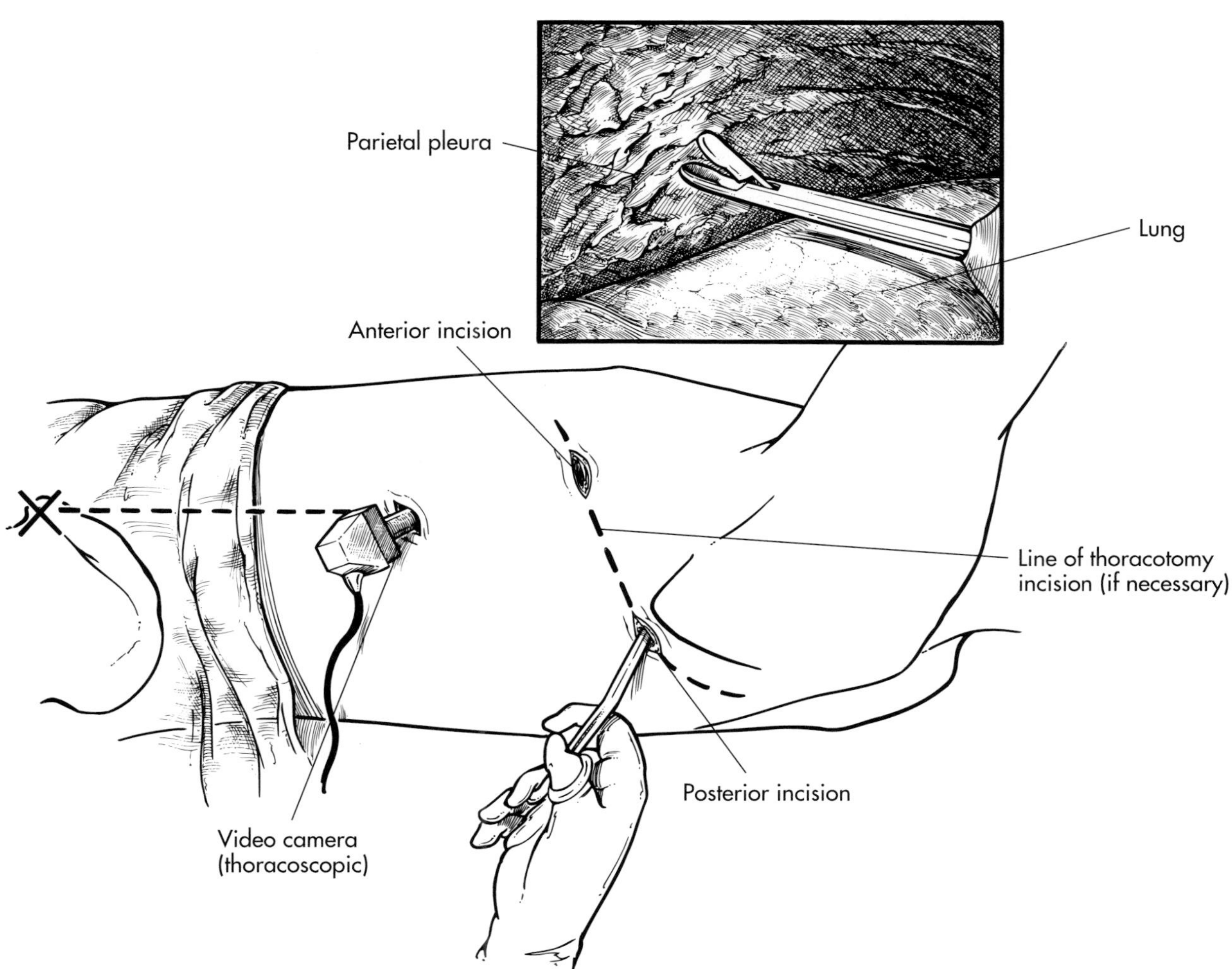
Parietal pleura
Lung
Anterior incision
Line of thoracotomy incision (if necessary)
Posterior incision
Video camera (thoracoscopic)

FIGURE 8-1

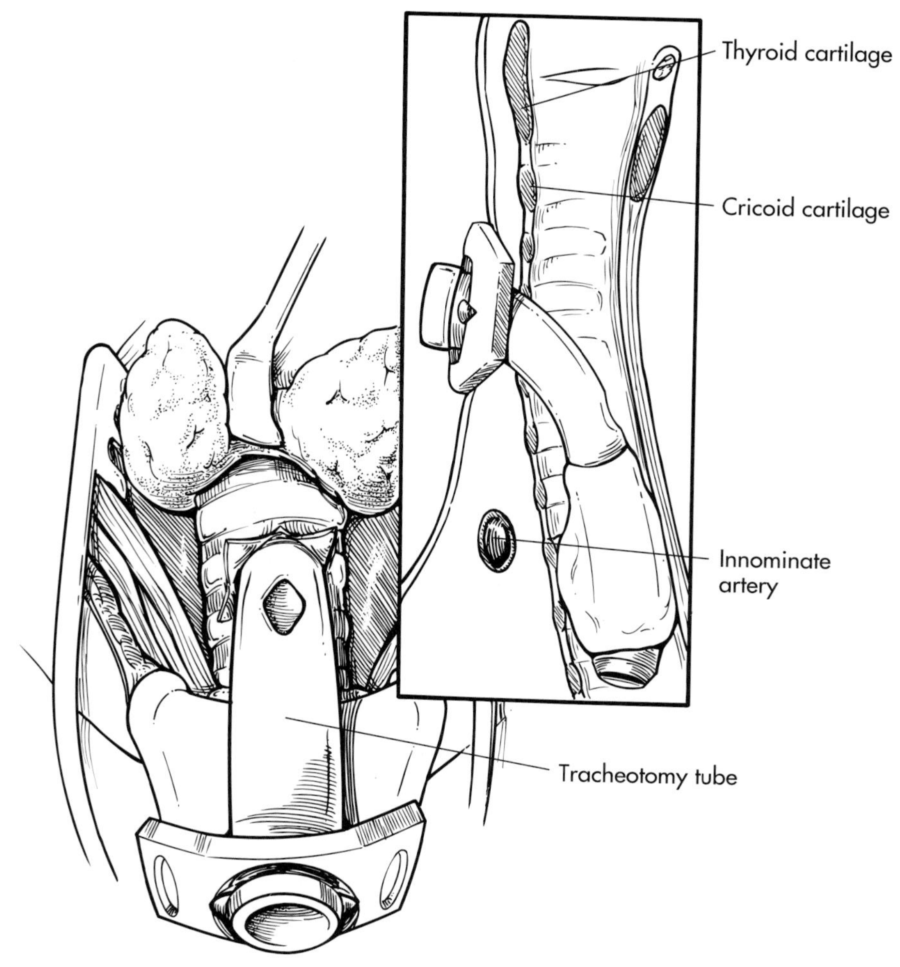

FIGURE 9-3

the flap sutured to the dermis prior to tube insertion. Some surgeons prefer to place a monofilament absorbable suture on each side of the tracheal opening and bring these sutures out of the wound to be used in case the tube needs to be reinserted early in the postoperative course. This maneuver is especially useful in the obese patient with a broad neck. In my hands, a cruciate incision has worked well and I continue to favor it.

Complications that may result from tracheostomy include erosion into the innominate artery, destruction of cartilaginous rings with stricture formation at the insertion site, and ischemia and late stricture formation at the cuff site. The development of low-pressure cuffs has greatly reduced the incidence of long-term cuff sequelae. Other complications include superficial wound infection and mucus plugging of the tube. The tube should not be changed for at least one week and preferably not until 10 days after the procedure to give the tract a chance to become established. If the tracheostoma is not adherent to the dermis, the intubation site may disappear into the depths of the subcutaneous tissue on attempting to change the tube.

Bibliography

Hazard P, Jones C, and Benitone J: Comparative clinical trial of standard operative tracheostomy with percutaneous tracheostomy, *Crit Care Med* 19:1018–1024, 1991.

Lewis RJ: Tracheostomies. Indications, timing and complications, *Clin Chest Med* 13:137–149, 1992.

Tayal VS: Tracheostomies, *Emerg Med Clin North Am* 12:707–727, 1994.

PART III

Thoracic Incisions

CHAPTER 10

Posterolateral Thoracotomy Incision

The posterolateral thoracotomy incision is the standard thoracotomy incision that has withstood the test of time. It provides excellent access to the entire hemithorax and is quite versatile. Classically, the surgeon stands to the side that is being operated on, thus the right side for a right thoracotomy and vice versa. In fact, it often proves easier and more efficient for the surgeon to stand on the opposite side to that which is being operated on. Viewing the hilum from the opposite side provides a distinct advantage. Anyone who spends time teaching others how to do pulmonary surgery knows this little secret.

DESCRIPTION OF THE PROCEDURE

The patient is placed in a full lateral position with the arm abducted, elevated, and flexed at the elbow and supported by an armrest. The lateral position is maintained either by sandbags or preferentially by a support device that becomes rigid when suction is applied, the so-called beanbag. This device, when positioned correctly, acts as an axillary protector to keep the body weight distributed and prevents injury to the neurovascular bundle. A separate axillary roll may have to be used as necessary. The table may be flexed at the hips to maximize the space between the ribs. Pillows are placed between the legs, and the down leg is slightly flexed but the up leg kept straight. The skin incision is made approximately 2 to 3 cm below the scapular tip; the incision should never cross the scapula (**Fig. 10-1**). We use electrocautery to deepen the incision once the skin is cut. There is no need to coagulate individual skin bleeders if the surgeon and the assistant place a lap pad along the entire cut edge of the incision and exert traction as the incision is being deepened. The latissimus dorsi muscle is divided and small blood vessels coagulated as they are encountered. It is not necessary to mobilize the muscle and get underneath it since the division is readily facilitated by the surgeon and the assistant applying traction and countertraction to the muscle as it is divided. This allows for easy visualization of blood vessels within the muscle.

Once the latissimus dorsi muscle is divided, the areolar tissue posterior to the serratus anterior muscle is incised along the direction of the muscle down to the chest wall. The cut edge of the latissimus dorsi muscle is mobilized off the serratus muscle using electrocautery. This allows the serratus muscle to be fully mobilized and preserved or divided, as desired. Adequate exposure is obtained either way. If the serratus anterior muscle is not divided, the free edge may be temporarily sewn to the skin edge to retract it out of the field.

A rib may be taken, but this is not a necessity. I enter the chest routinely through the bed of the resected fifth rib or in the fifth intercostal space for all pulmonary surgery (**Fig. 10-2**); the location of the hilum is constant no matter whether one is doing an upper or a lower lobectomy. I see no advantage to going through the sixth intercostal space unless one is performing an esophagectomy. The scapula is retracted superiorly, allowing access to the fifth rib, which is obscured by the scapula. The

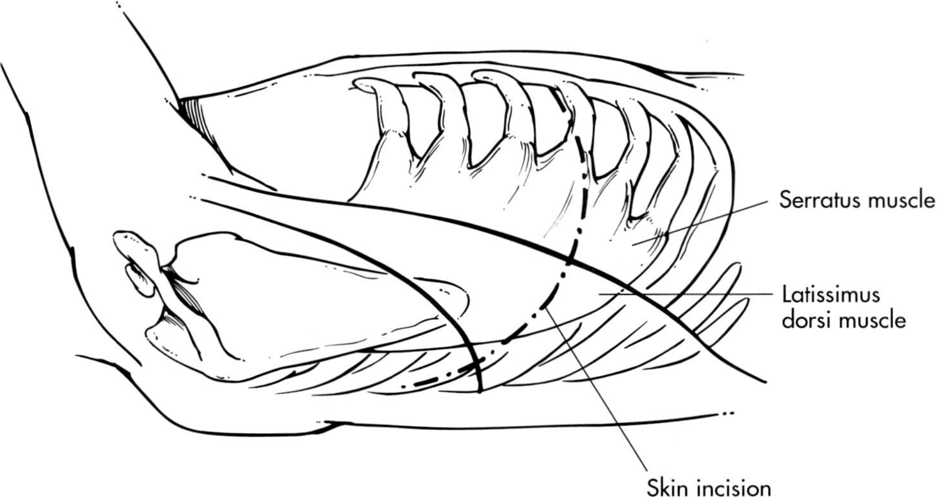

FIGURE 10-1

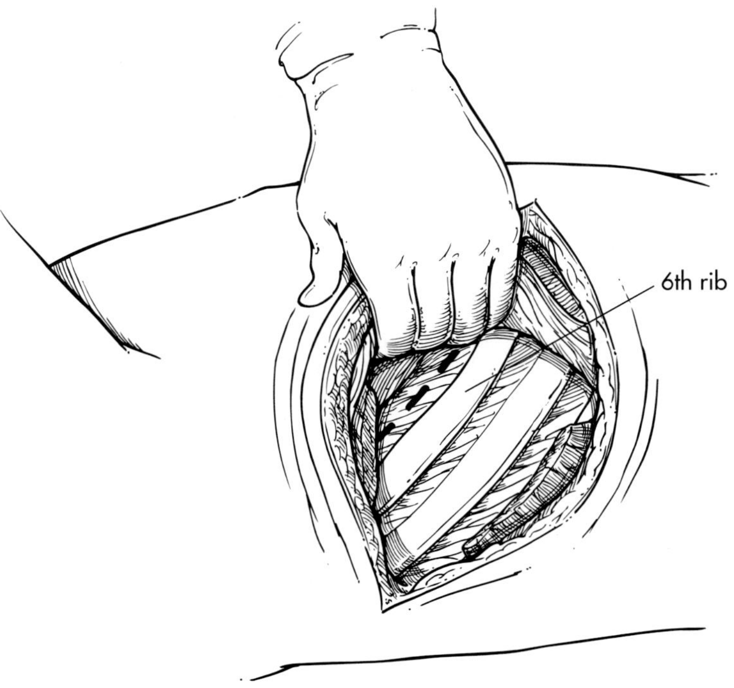

FIGURE 10-2

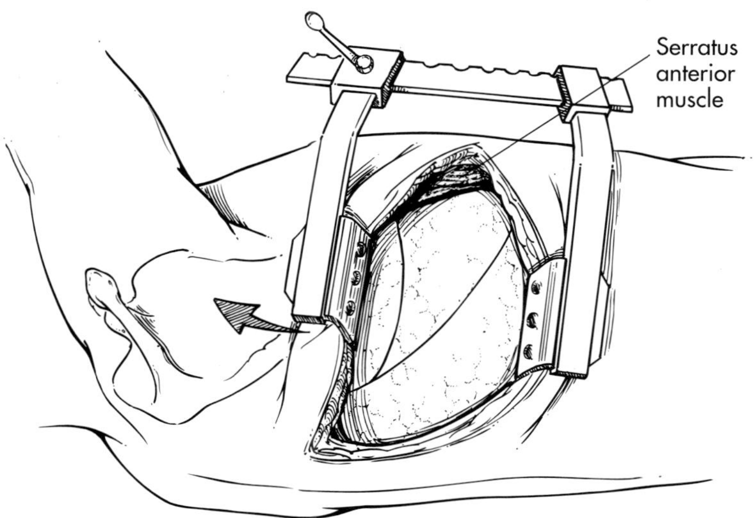

FIGURE 10-3

sixth rib is usually the first one not obscured by the scapula. The ribs are counted by placing a hand underneath (anterior) the scapula and reaching up posteriorly to identify the posterior scalene as it inserts on the second rib. This is a consistent anatomic finding and always identifies the second rib. It is sometimes difficult to reach all the way up to the first rib, which can result in an inaccurate rib count and entry in the wrong space. The intercostal space between the second and third ribs is usually wider than the other spaces, which aids identification. Excision of the rib proceeds in a subperiosteal fashion by first incising the periosteum overlying the rib and stripping it off superiorly and inferiorly. A Doyenne or Matson elevator is used to strip the periosteum from the medial portion of the rib. The rib is cut and removed. Alternatively, the chest is entered by dividing the intercostal muscle at the superior edge of the sixth rib, going as far posterior as the anterior edge of the erector spinae ligament. A small piece, 2 to 3 cm, of the posterior sixth rib may be taken, which allows the rib to move more easily when the rib spreader is opened and may prevent rib fracture.

A rib spreader is placed and slowly opened to avoid breaking a rib, which causes additional morbidity from increased postoperative pain (**Fig. 10-3**). The intercostal space is spread only as much as necessary to accomplish the operative procedure; the less the space is spread, the less the postoperative pain.

The incision is closed by placing heavy sutures around the fifth and sixth ribs, so-called pericostal sutures. The ribs are brought together either by the assistant's pulling on an adjacent, not yet tied, suture or by placing a rib approximator (Bailey). If a rib has been removed, the intercostal muscle should be reapproximated with a continuous absorbable suture. The serratus anterior muscle, if it has been divided, and the fibrofatty tissue posterior to the serratus are closed, and the latissimus dorsi muscle edges are sutured. The skin is closed with a running subcuticular suture (preferably) or skin staples.

Bibliography

Fry WA: Thoracic incisions. In Shields TW, ed: *General thoracic surgery*, Philadelphia, 1994, Williams & Wilkins.

Ponn RB, Ferneini A, D'Agostino RS, et al: Comparison of late pulmonary function after posterolateral and muscle-sparing thoracotomy, *Ann Thorac Surg* 53:675–679, 1992.

C H A P T E R 11

Vertical Axillary (Muscle-Sparing) Thoracotomy Incision

There is no question that the posterolateral thoracotomy incision has withstood the test of time and is the "standard" thoracotomy incision used today. This incision is large, frequently results in rib fractures, and at the very least divides the latissimus dorsi muscle and usually the serratus anterior muscle as well. There are several muscle-sparing alternatives that have been described, and we favor one that starts with a vertical axillary skin incision. We use this standard thoracotomy incision for all chest procedures, except those in which chest wall resection is likely unless the area of chest wall to be resected is anterior. Otherwise, we have used the incision for all other lung lesions, redo thoracotomies, esophageal operations, posterior mediastinal lesions, and exposure of thoracic vertebral bodies. The exposure provided is excellent, as good as that obtained with the posterolateral incision, and patient acceptance is better. Return of upper extremity function is quicker, and the patients are more satisfied with the cosmetic aspects of the incision. No skin or muscle flaps are raised; thus seromas or hematomas have not been seen.

DESCRIPTION OF THE PROCEDURE

The patient is placed in the lateral decubitus position with the ipsilateral arm maximally abducted and flexed at the elbow. The skin incision is placed just posterior to the lateral edge of the pectoral is major muscle and extends for approximately 6 cm (**Fig. 11-1**). It is placed slightly farther posteriorly

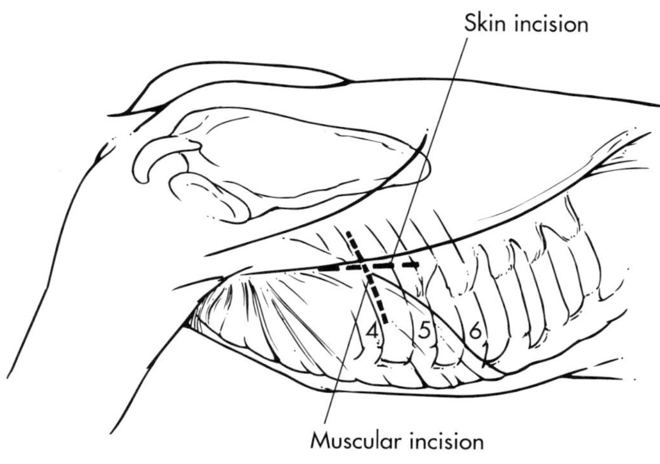

FIGURE 11-1

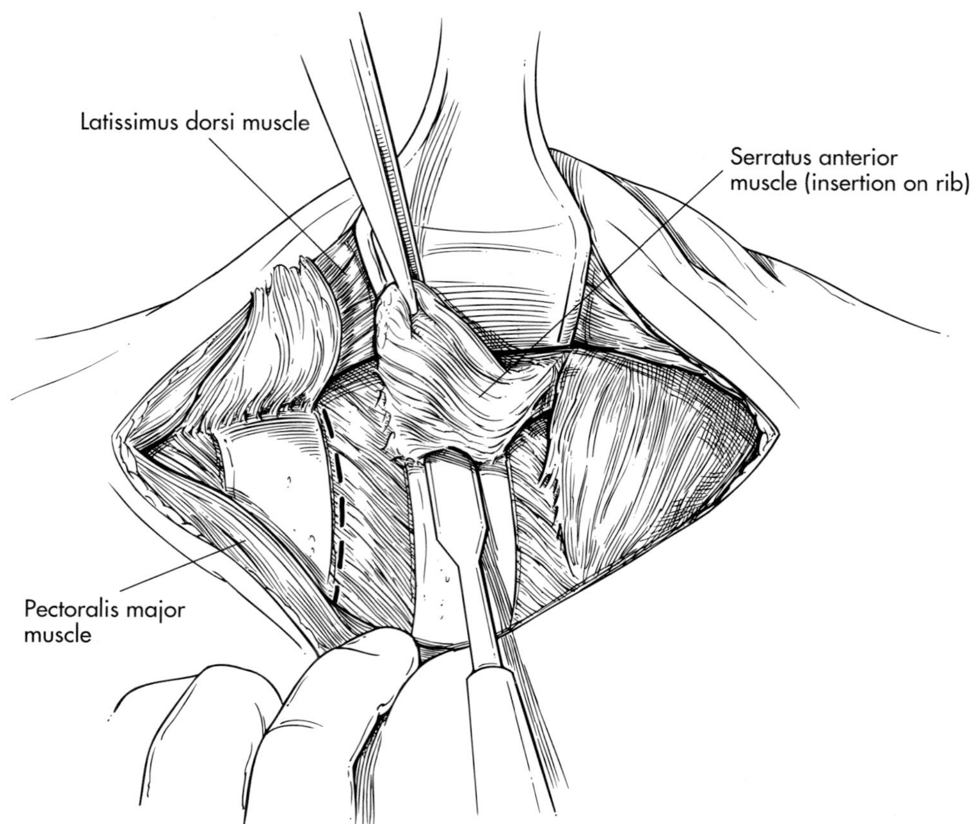

FIGURE 11-2

in women to avoid the added downward traction exerted postoperatively on the healing wound by the breast. Upon deepening of the incision through the subcutaneous tissue, the lateral border of the pectoralis is mobilized and undermined to free it posteriorly off the chest wall (**Fig. 11-2**). Since this incision is somewhat more anterior than the standard posterolateral incision, the chest is entered through the fourth intercostal space rather than the fifth. The insertions of the serratus anterior muscle on the fourth and fifth ribs are freed from the ribs and reflected posteriorly (***see*** **Fig. 11-2**). No muscle is divided. Freeing the insertions of the serratus muscle exposes the fourth intercostal space, which is incised along the superior aspect of the fifth rib. A rib spreader is inserted, and from inside the chest the intercostal incision is extended as far posteriorly as possible (**Fig. 11-3**). The full thickness of the intercostal muscles is divided, but the overlying latissimus dorsi and serratus anterior muscle are preserved. The rib spreader is opened as wide as necessary for exposure, and a Balfour retractor is placed perpendicularly to retract the skin and muscle (**Fig. 11-4**). The Balfour retractor is opened widely, which allows for excellent exposure of all intrathoracic structures. The more anterior location of the incision gives better access to the hilum than afforded by the posterolateral approach. Rarely does rib fracture occur with rib spreading because of the extent of the intercostal incision achieved by opening from within.

The incision is closed with heavy paracostal sutures to reapproximate the ribs, and the freed insertions of the serratus muscle are sutured medially. The subcutaneous tissue is reapproximated and the skin closed as usual.

Because of the short length of the incision, the slightly deeper hole mandates the use of a headlight (standard equipment for the thoracic surgeon), requires the lung to be retracted with a gauze

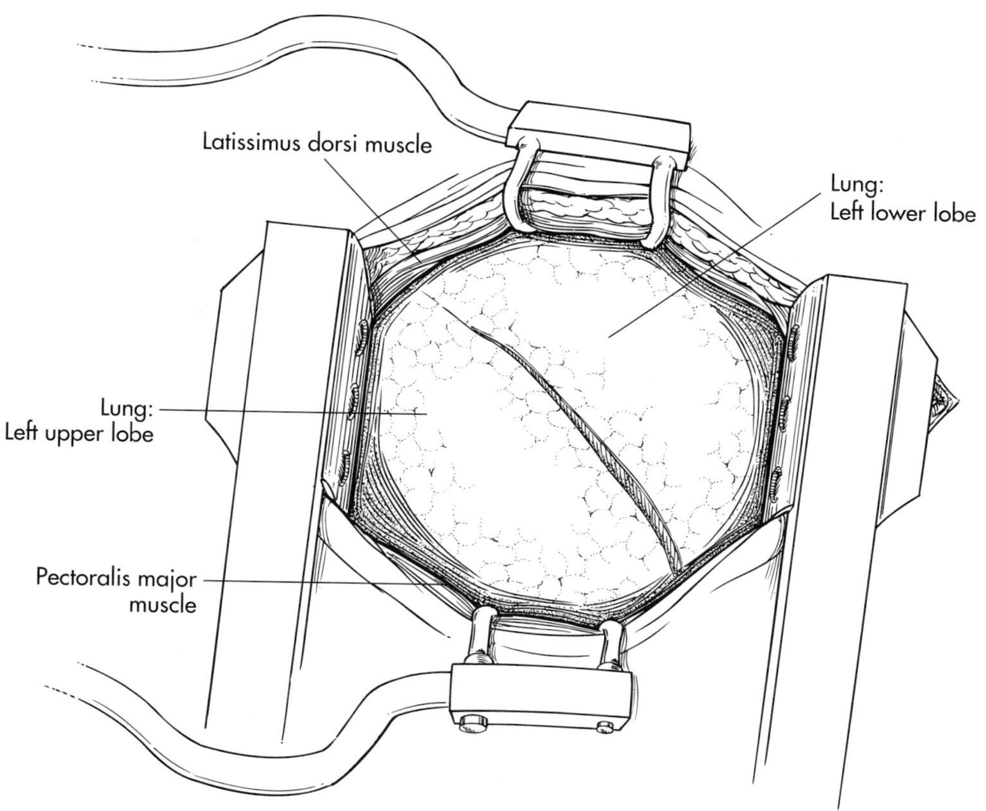

FIGURE 11-3

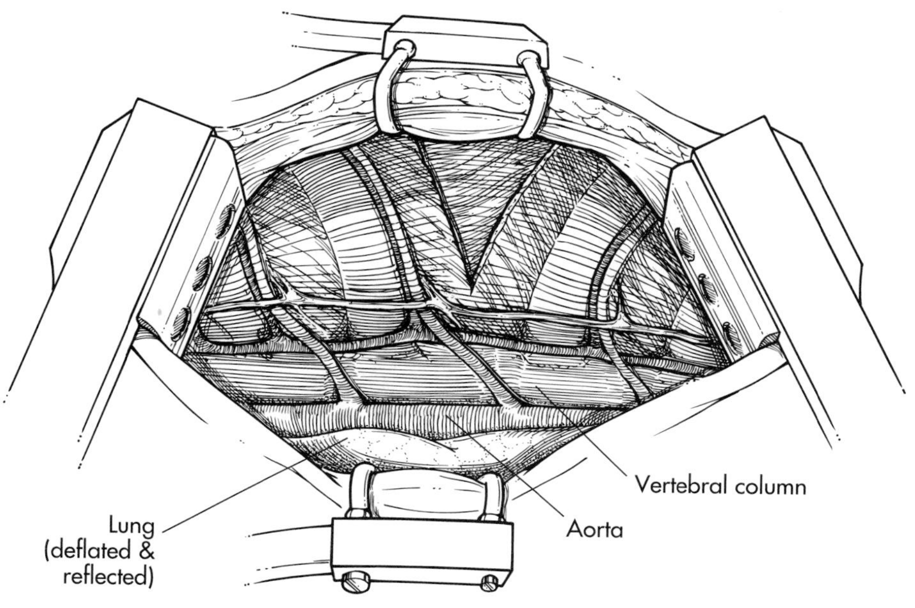

FIGURE 11-4

on a sponge holder rather than the hand, and makes stapler placement slightly more difficult because of the angles created by the increased depth.

The only difficulties encountered have been related to placement of the skin incision. If the incision is placed too far anteriorly in women, the weight of the breast has caused some widening of the incision and an occasional separation that has been allowed to granulate. In the obese patient, the skin folds in the axilla can cause maceration of the incision with resultant partial separation.

Bibliography

Bethencourt DM, Holmes EC: Muscle sparing posterolateral thoracotomy, *Ann Thorac Surg* 45:337–339, 1988.

Ginsberg RJ: Alternative (muscle-sparing) incisions in thoracic surgery, *Ann Thorac Surg* 56:752–754, 1993.

Hayward RH, Knight WL, Baisden CE, et al: Access to the thorax by incision, *J Am Coll Surg* 179:202–208, 1994.

Hazelrigg SR, Landreneau RL, Boley TM, et al: The effect of muscle-sparing versus standard posterolateral thoracotomy on pulmonary function, muscle strength, and postoperative pain, *J Thorac Cardiovasc Surg* 101:394–400, 1991.

Mitchell RL: The lateral limited thoracotomy incision: standard for pulmonary operations, *J Thorac Cardiovasc Surg* 91:1259–1264, 1990.

CHAPTER 12

Median Sternotomy Incision

The median sternotomy incision is the standard incision used for heart surgery, but it has taken on an increased role in pulmonary surgery over the past few years. The incision seems to result in less postoperative pain than an intercostal incision and thus has found new utility in procedures performed on patients with borderline pulmonary function. Access to both hemithoraces is permitted by this incision, yet exposure is difficult, especially posteriorly, if significant adhesions must be lysed. Bilateral lung volume reduction operations are performed using this incision, which avoids rib spreading and the resultant postoperative pain. Anatomic pulmonary resections on patients with borderline pulmonary function may also be performed through this incision. Because of the heart, left lower lobectomy presents a significant challenge through this approach. Median sternotomy is also useful for exposure of the origin of the innominate artery after penetrating chest trauma and for resection of anterior mediastinal tumors.

DESCRIPTION OF THE PROCEDURE

The patient is placed on the operating table in the supine position. A skin incision is made from the sternal notch to just inferior to the xiphoid process (**Fig. 12-1**). The subcutaneous tissue is divided with electrocautery, and the periosteum overlying the midportion of the sternum is incised. There is a ligamentous attachment on the posterior aspect of the sternal notch that must be divided, and a finger is inserted posterior to the notch to free the posterior aspect of the sternum. The pleural reflections are swept laterally. If the saw is placed at the sternal notch and drawn downward, there is no need to dissect around the xiphoid process. Placing the saw inferiorly and going toward the notch requires finger dissection posterior to the xiphoid to free up the posterior sternum.

A reciprocating sternal saw is used to divide the sternum. The lungs should be deflated before placing the saw to avoid cutting a pleural reflection (**Fig. 12-2**). There usually is considerable bleeding initially from the cut sternal edges, and electrocautery is used on the incised periosteum. I try to avoid using bone wax, which may contribute to delayed wound healing. A sternal retractor is placed and slowly opened only as wide as necessary, since brachial plexus injury can result from opening the sternum too widely. For some pulmonary procedures it may be advantageous to use a hemisternal retractor, which lefts on the sternal edge anteriorly for enhanced exposure of a pleural space.

The sternotomy incision is closed by first placing wires through the sternum. I place two wires through the manubrium and at least four wires in the body of the sternum. The wires may be placed around the sternum or through the bone, but care should be taken to avoid the internal mammary artery. The wires are twisted and secured to approximate the sternal edges. Absorbable sutures are used to reapproximate the pectoralis major muscle in the midline, the subcutaneous tissue is sutured, and the skin is closed.

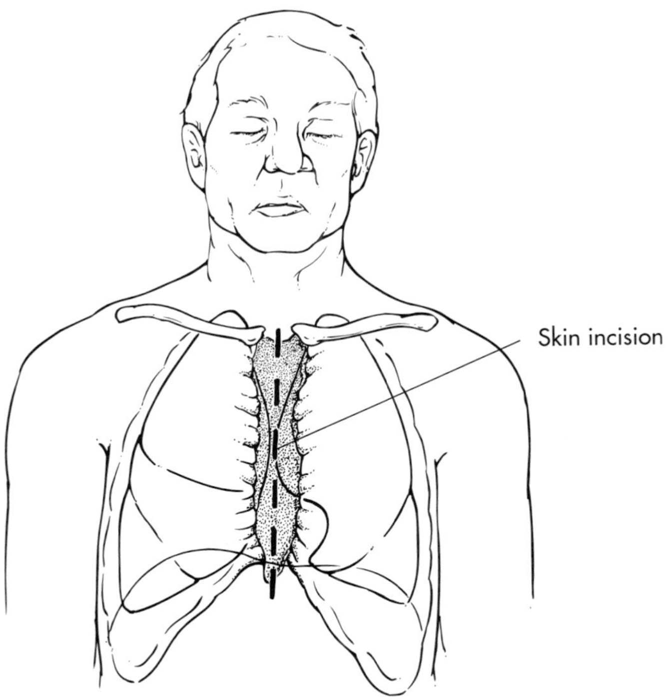

FIGURE 12-1

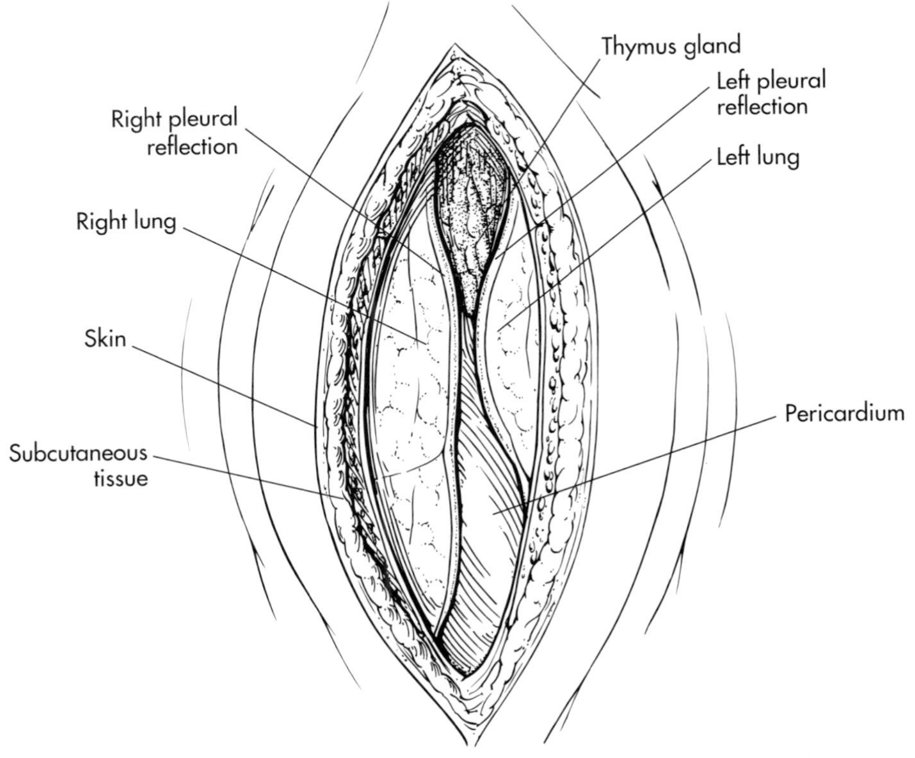

FIGURE 12-2

Bibliography

Bains MS, Ginsberg RJ, Jones WG II, et al: The clamshell incision: an improved approach to bilateral pulmonary and mediastinal tumors, *Ann Thorac Surg* 58:30–32, 1994.

Pasque MK, Cooper JD, Kaiser LR, et al: Improved technique for bilateral lung transplantation: rationale and initial clinical experience, *Ann Thorac Surg* 49:785–791, 1990.

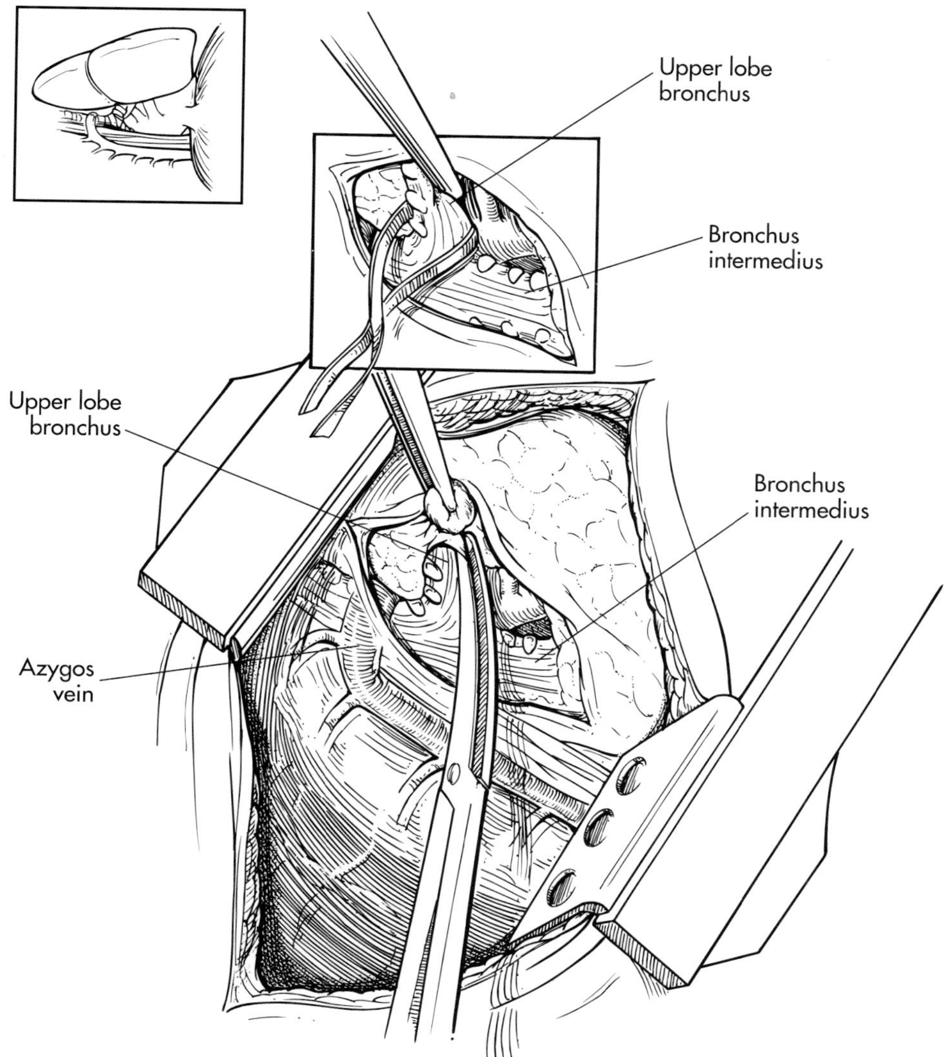

FIGURE 14-4

firing a stapler across the fissure adds little; it really brings one no closer to the artery. Taking advantage of the anatomy posteriorly allows easy identification of the artery in the fissure without actually dissecting in the fissure. It is important to remember that the fissure is defined by the artery. Once the artery is identified and dissected the posterior portion of the major fissure is very easy to complete (see **Fig. 14-5**).

Alternatively, the upper lobe bronchus may be encircled and divided at this point which allows complete visualization of the artery from "behind" the fissure. This is the preferable move when there is nodal involvement in the fissure that makes dissection of the artery difficult. The arterial branch to the posterior segment of the upper lobe is adjacent (superior) to the superior segmental branch and at times may arise from this branch (**Fig. 14-6**). The arterial supply to the middle lobe usually arises just opposite the takeoff of the superior segmental branch. There is usually one middle lobe branch, but two branches are not uncommon.

The lung is again retracted posteriorly and the vascular structures divided now that the entire resection has been laid out. I rarely divide any structure before getting a complete "lay of the land". Resectability must be assured before dividing any vascular structures. The arterial branch to the anterior and apical segments is divided between ligatures, preferably silk. If tumor or nodal involvement

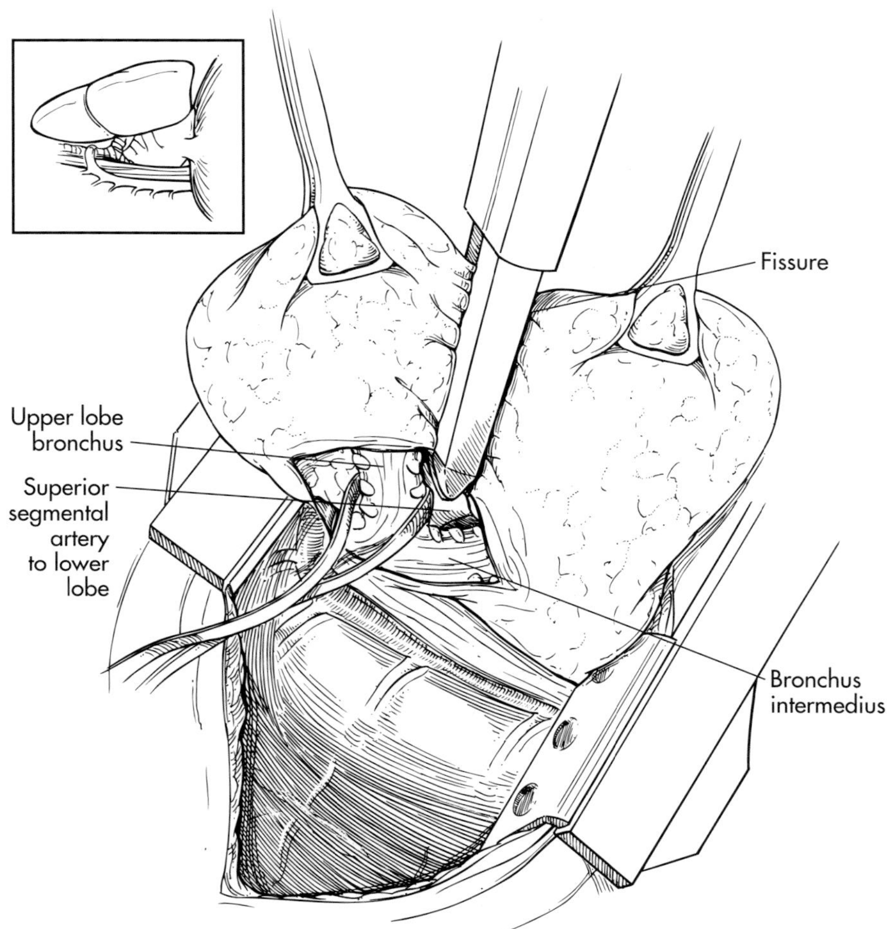
Fissure
Upper lobe bronchus
Superior segmental artery to lower lobe
Bronchus intermedius

FIGURE 14-5

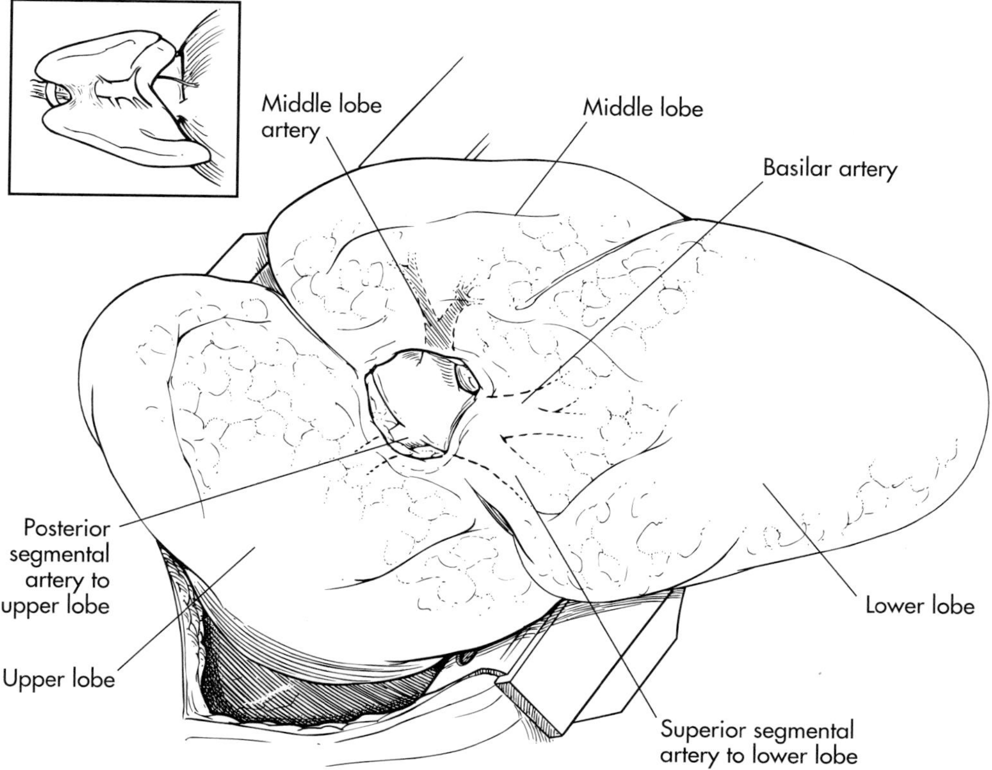

FIGURE 14-6

obscures the takeoff of the anterior-apical trunk, instead of trying to dissect in this area it is often simpler to snug down the Rumel tourniquet on the proximal pulmonary artery, encircle the artery distally in the fissure with a vessel loop, and either cut the arterial branch or resect a portion of the arterial wall where the tumor is adherent or invading. The artery is then repaired with a running 6-0 monofilament nonabsorbable suture. Even with proximal and distal control some back bleeding occurs, but it is not particularly troublesome. I do not hesitate to take arterial branches in this way when there is tumor present that precludes safe dissection around an arterial branch. It is often easier to get proximal and distal to a problem area, then divide and repair. At times a significantly large portion of the anterior arterial wall must be taken, and a patch may be necessary to preserve the luminal diameter of the artery. In these situations we harvest a piece of pericardium and use this as an onlay patch graft. Once the arterial trunk is divided, the origin of the upper lobe bronchus may be seen from this anterior approach. Lymph nodes lying along the bronchus are dissected distally to be removed with the specimen. Often, this node will be the same as that seen posteriorly when the crotch between the upper lobe bronchus and bronchus intermedius was dissected. Freeing these nodes completes the dissection around the bronchus.

The superior pulmonary vein is divided between lines of staples laid down by a vascular stapler but alternatively the vein may be ligated, then suture ligated to assure safety (**Fig. 14-7**). A vascular clamp may also be placed and the divided vein sutured with a horizontal mattress stitch, the clamp removed, and the suture run as a simple stitch anterior to the mattress stitch back to where it was begun and then tied. Once the vein is divided, the continuation of the artery is identified as it lies posterior to the vein. The middle lobe arterial branch is readily identified from the anterior aspect of the hilum and, to facilitate division of the fissure and separation of the middle lobe from the upper lobe, the branch should be dissected for a short distance. The arterial branch to the posterior segment of the upper lobe at times may be seen through this anterior exposure, or an additional anterior segmental branch may be identified. Once the artery is identified from this anterior approach and the

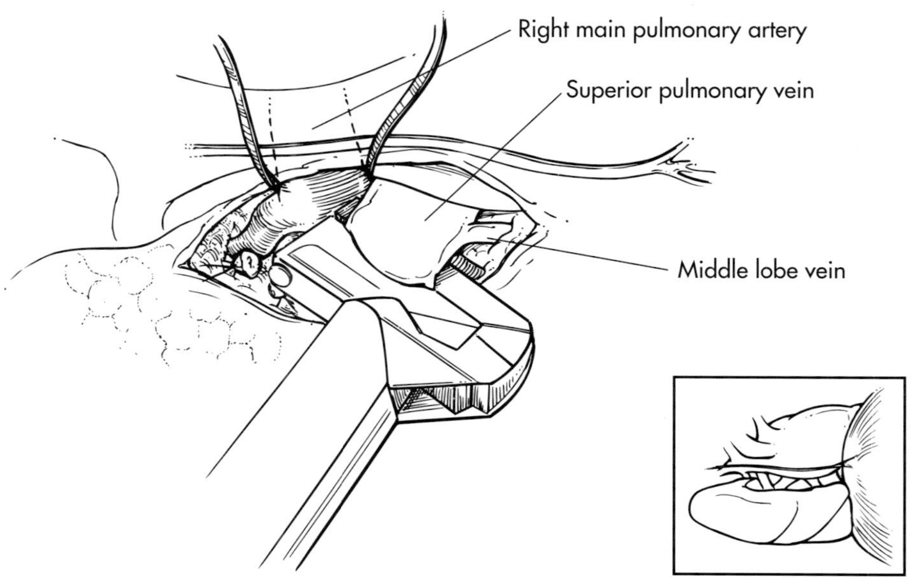

FIGURE 14-7

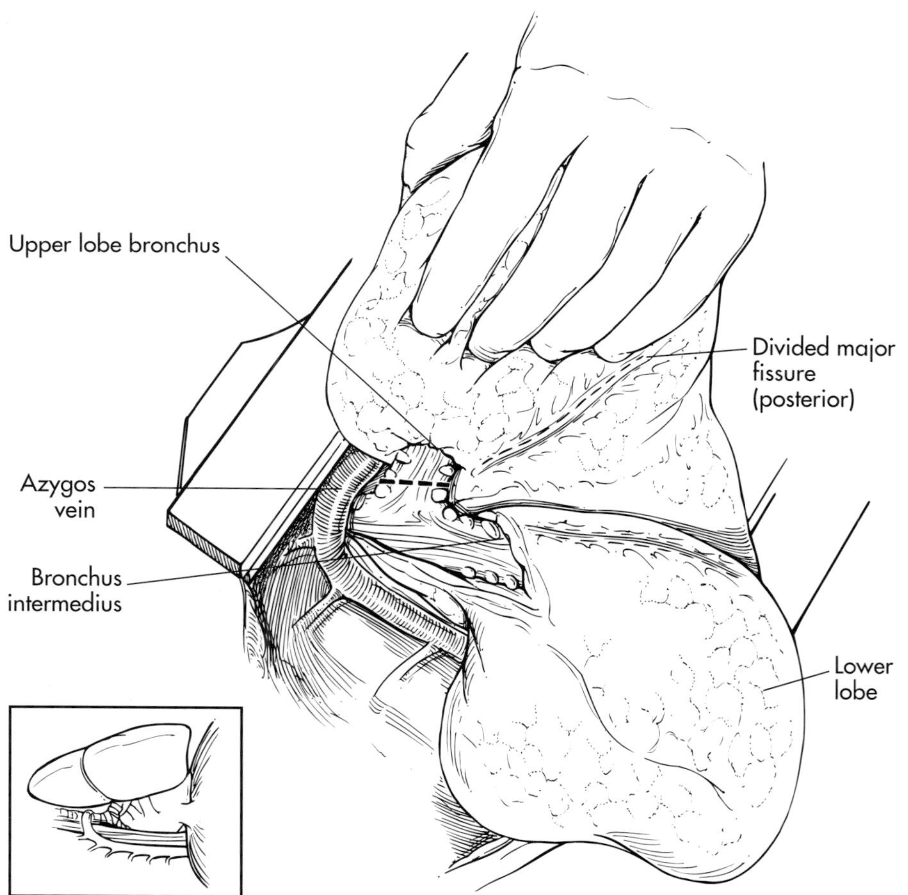

FIGURE 14-8

middle lobe artery is seen, the minor fissure, which is usually incomplete and poorly formed, may be divided with an application of the linear stapler. Often I save this division of the minor fissure until after I have divided the bronchus and it is the only thing holding the upper lobe in place.

The posterior segmental branch of the artery is ligated and divided within the fissure. With the lung again retracted anteriorly, the origin of the upper lobe bronchus is well seen and a stapler is placed and fired (**Fig. 14-8**). The bronchus is taken as close as possible to its origin but without compromising the right main bronchus. With the dissection performed as described, any problem with the main bronchus should be easily avoided. The bronchus is divided and the upper lobe removed if the minor fissure has been divided. If the minor fissure remains, it is completed with a firing of the linear stapler. To obtain definitive staging information the surgeon performs a mediastinal lymph node dissection.

After division of the minor fissure and removal of the right upper lobe, the middle lobe is left without much support since the oblique fissure usually is complete. This situation may predispose to torsion and infarction of the middle lobe in the postoperative period. To prevent this very significant complication the surgeon "re-attaches" the middle lobe to the lower lobe either by placing one or two absorbable sutures in a figure-of-eight pattern or by firing a linear stapler from which the blade has been removed. Care must be taken to assure that the middle lobe is properly oriented before attaching it to the lower lobe.

Bibliography

Hayward RH, Knight WL, Baisden CE, et al: Access to the thorax by incision, *J Am Coll Surg* 179:202–208, 1994.

CHAPTER 15

Right Middle Lobectomy

Middle lobectomy is thought by many to be the most difficult lobectomy because of the problems presented by the fissures. This is an erroneous concept, and I will present two ways to accomplish this lobectomy, the choice of technique being dependent on the status of the fissures. As illustrated here, the procedure is being performed through a vertical axillary muscle-sparing incision (**Fig. 15-1**). Briefly, the incision is made just posterior to the pectoralis major muscle and carried down to the chest wall. The pectoralis muscle is undermined anteriorly, and the insertions of the serratus anterior muscle on ribs 4 and 5 are freed off the rib and reflected posteriorly without dividing any of the muscle. The chest is entered through the fourth intercostal space, and the rib spreader is inserted. The intercostal incision is carried as far posterior as possible by completing the division of the intercostal musculature from within the chest. A Balfour abdominal retractor is placed perpendicular to the rib spreader to retract the skin edges. The combination of the two retractors provides excellent exposure to the entire chest and its contents.

DESCRIPTION OF THE PROCEDURE

The illustrations depict the view from the left side of the table, the ideal position from which to operate through this incision. If the major fissure is well developed and the pulmonary artery can be visualized easily within the fissure, the dissection is begun over the pulmonary artery. If the artery is not

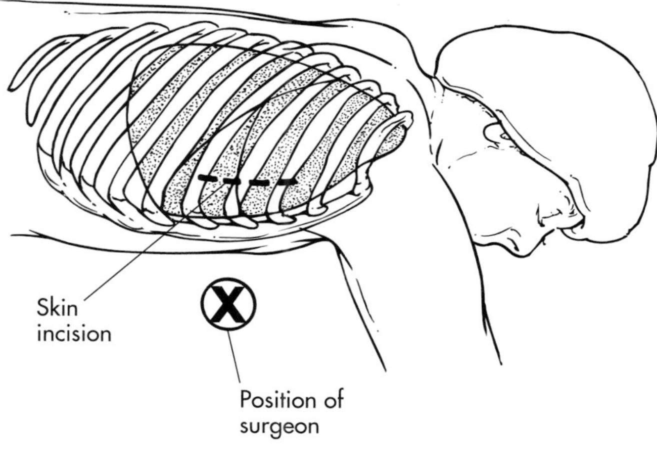

FIGURE 15-1

CHAPTER 16

Right Lower Lobectomy

Because of the close proximity of the bronchovascular structures of the middle lobe, resection of the right lower lobe provides several unique challenges and is one of the more difficult lobectomies. As in the middle lobectomy, the pulmonary artery must be identified within the fissure to complete the resection, and in those cases where the fissure is poorly developed a direct attack through parenchyma often proves to be quite challenging. The chest is entered through either a standard posterolateral thoracotomy incision (5th intercostal space) or a vertical axillary muscle-sparing incision (4th space). **Figure 16-1** illustrates the placement of the vertical axillary incision. The drawings illustrate the view from the left side of the table, which is the ideal side from which to work. If disease is noted within the fissure or if the hilum is involved, it is best to obtain control of the proximal right main pulmonary artery. The hilar pleura is incised anteriorly and superiorly, with the lung retracted in a posterior direction by the surgeon. The right main pulmonary artery is encircled with a finger after the appropriate plane of dissection is entered. An umbilical tape is passed and a Rumel tourniquet placed.

If the fissure is reasonably well developed, the pleura overlying the pulmonary artery is incised and the dissection is carried down onto the plane of the artery (**Fig. 16-2**). The branch to the superior segment of the lower lobe is first identified, and the middle lobe branch is most commonly found arising from the opposite aspect of the artery just across from the superior segmental origin. The dissection may be extended posteriorly along the superior aspect of the branch to the superior segment that leads to the bifurcation of the upper lobe bronchus and bronchus intermedius. With the lung retracted anteriorly, the pleura overlying this bifurcation posteriorly is incised and a linear stapler may be inserted from just above the superior segmental arterial branch through the area of the bifurcation (**Fig. 16-3**). This move is possible since there are no vascular structures present posterior to the

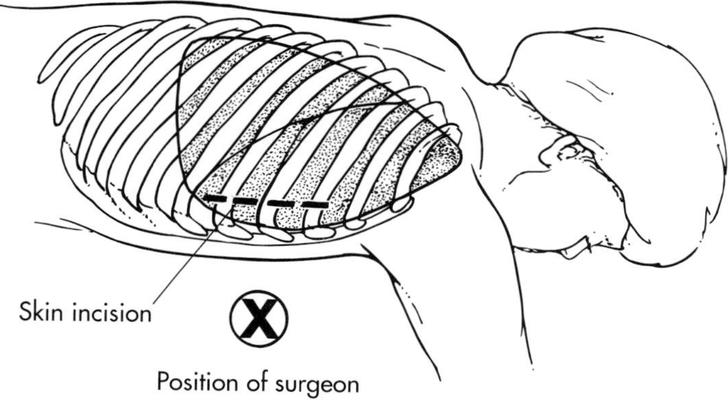

FIGURE 16-1

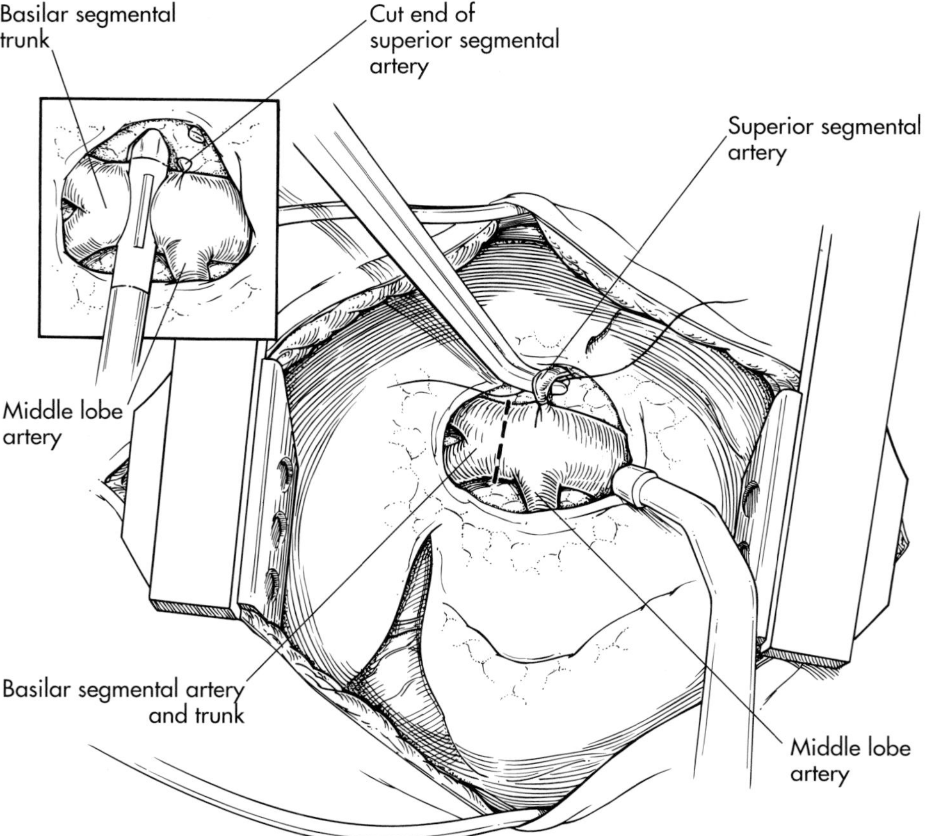

FIGURE 16-2

origin of the superior segmental arterial branch. On the superior aspect of the artery just across from the superior segment, the posterior segmental branch, the so-called "recurrent" branch, to the upper lobe arises and is easily visualized. Rarely this branch to the upper lobe may arise from the superior segmental branch to the lower lobe, but this possibility should be kept in mind. The posterior aspect of the major fissure is then divided and completed. Completing the posterior aspect of the fissure at this point allows more room to work on the artery, making the dissection safer.

The relationship of the superior segmental branch to the middle lobe arterial branch determines whether the lower lobe artery may be divided as a complete trunk or whether the superior segmental branch and basilar trunk need to be taken separately. As illustrated in **Figure 16-2**, the superior segmental branch must be taken separately to avoid damage to the middle lobe arterial supply. The dotted line indicates the position for division of the basilar segmental trunk. This is usually a 1- to 2-cm trunk and should be double ligated with a suture ligature or, as we prefer, closed with a vascular stapler, then divided. The simplest stapling maneuver utilizes the endoscopic linear stapler with a vascular cartridge (**Fig. 16-2, *inset***). This lays down three parallel rows of staples on each side of the blade, and I have found this to be a safe, reliable maneuver.

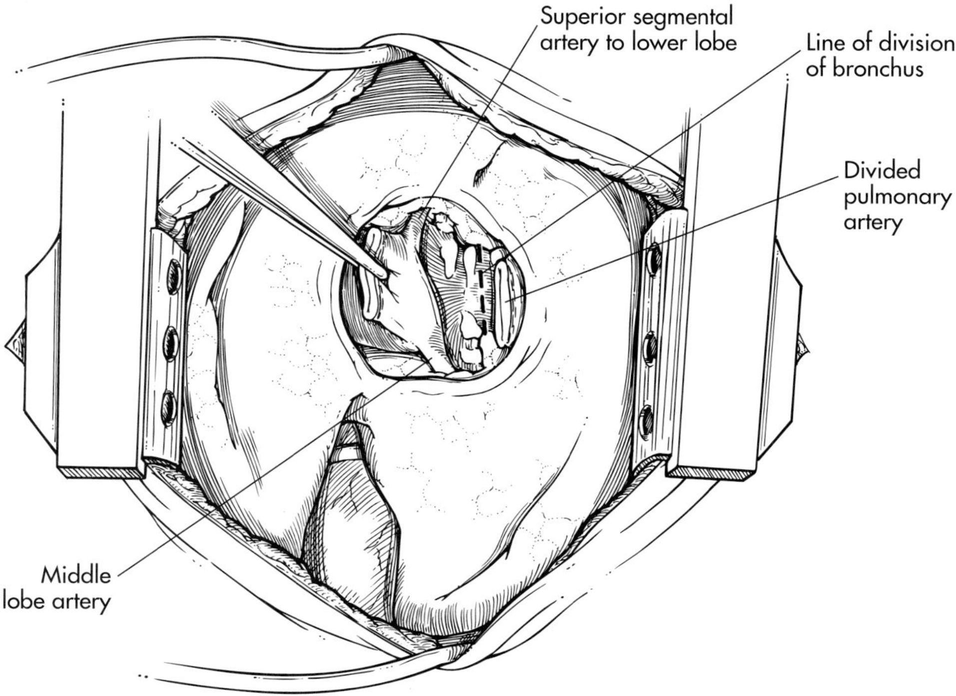

FIGURE 16-7

the upper lobe bronchus is at somewhat increased risk for breakdown compared to other bronchial closures.

Lesions within the bronchus intermedius often present additional problems for the surgeon. These lesions often involve the superior pulmonary vein, occasionally with proximal extension into the left atrium. Careful exploration is mandated to assess resectability before dividing any structures. Proximal involvement of the inferior pulmonary vein need not preclude resection if the vessel can be encircled or the extent of atrial involvement is not excessive. Some of these lesions may demand intrapericardial pneumonectomy because of the proximal involvement of the atrium.

Bibliography

Keller SM, Kaiser LR, and Martini N: Bilobectomy for bronchogenic carcinoma, *Ann Thorac Surg* 45:62–65, 1988.

C H A P T E R 17

Right Pneumonectomy

Right pneumonectomy, from a technical standpoint, is a relatively simple and usually straightforward procedure but the complications that may result from total removal of the right lung are anything but simple or easy to manage. Right pneumonectomy should be performed only when alternative resections, including bronchoplastic procedures, are not feasible. Lesions that mandate pneumonectomy are mainly those that involve the very proximal pulmonary artery or larger lesions that arise within the center of the lung and involve all three lobes. Most commonly, it is proximal involvement of the artery that is responsible for pneumonectomy. A "difficult" fissure should not be an indication for pneumonectomy. Relative contraindications to pneumonectomy include baseline pulmonary function that would leave inadequate pulmonary reserve after resection, inability to remove all disease, and advanced age.

A quantitative perfusion lung scan should be performed to assess relative blood flow to each lung if the FEV_1 is less than 2 L. It is not surprising that even patients with borderline lung function are candidates for pneumonectomy because of relatively little perfusion going to the lung proposed for resection. In a sense, some of these patients are already "autopneumonectomized."

Lung conservation should always be kept in mind at the start of any pulmonary resection, and it is only the rare resection that I begin knowing that I will have to perform pneumonectomy. Most commonly, the decision to remove the entire lung is made intraoperatively after thorough exploration of the chest and assessment of the extent of the lesion. Sometimes the surgeon carries this assessment so far as to begin performing the resection as if lobectomy or sleeve lobectomy is possible and converting to pneumonectomy only when a lesser resection proves to be impossible to complete.

DESCRIPTION OF THE PROCEDURE

The chest is entered through either a standard posterolateral thoracotomy incision (5th intercostal space) (**Fig. 17-1**), or a vertical axillary muscle-sparing incision (4th space). With a bronchoplastic procedure or pneumonectomy a possibility, the anesthesiologist will have placed the double-lumen endobronchial tube in the bronchus opposite to the side being operated. In this case, a left endobronchial tube would have been placed. It is the surgeon's responsibility to convey the nature of the possible resection to the anesthesiologist so that the appropriate double-lumen tube is placed. The lung is retracted posteriorly by the surgeon to expose the anterior hilum where the pleura is incised, carrying this superiorly over the bronchus and inferiorly to the level of the inferior pulmonary vein (**Fig. 17-2**). The inferior pulmonary ligament is incised up to the level of the inferior vein and the vein is encircled. The right main pulmonary artery is identified, as is the superior pulmonary vein. The artery is followed proximally to where it courses medial to the vena cava. After entering the appropriate dissection plane, the surgeon encircles the proximal pulmonary artery with a finger.

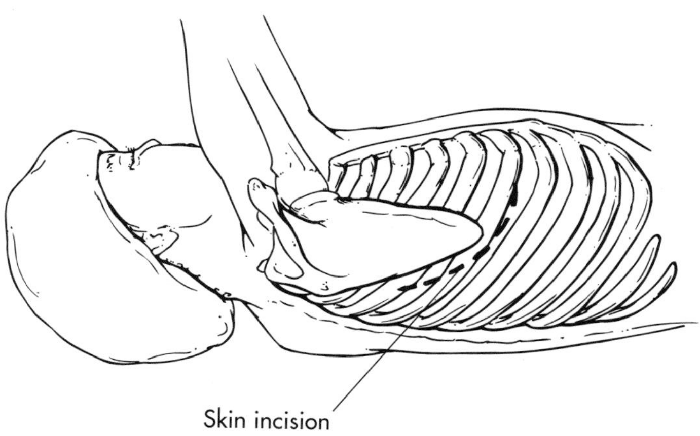

FIGURE 17-1

Main pulmonary artery

Superior pulmonary vein

Right main pulmonary artery

Inferior pulmonary vein

Superior pulmonary vein

Middle lobe vein

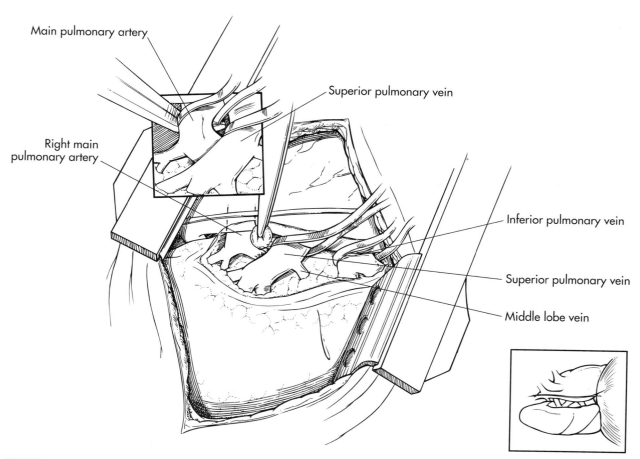

FIGURE 17-2

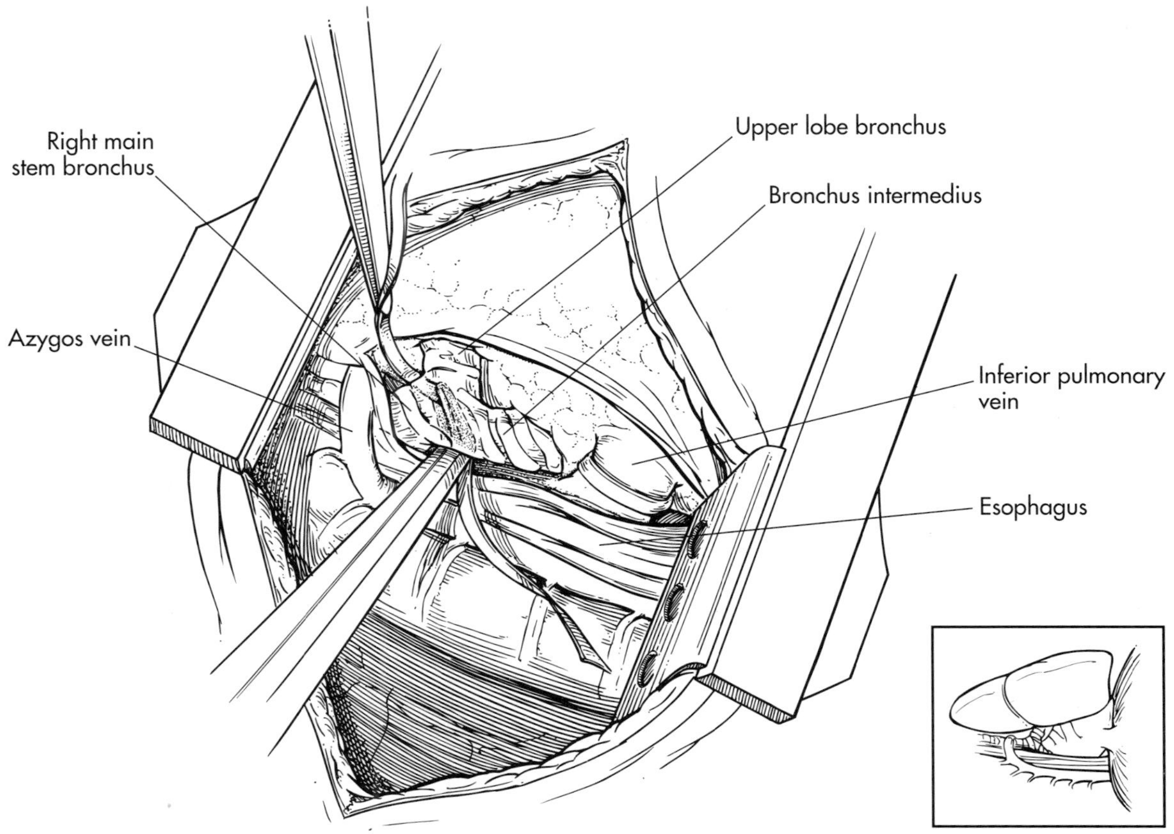

FIGURE 17-3

The superior pulmonary vein is dissected and encircled. Care must be taken to avoid injury to the continuation of the pulmonary artery as it courses medial to the superior pulmonary vein. The plane between these two vessels must be entered to separate them (**Fig. 17-2, *inset***). With a proximal tumor encasing the hilum, usually it is necessary to open the pericardium to fully assess resectability and control the vessels. Opening the pericardium allows for an assessment of mediastinal invasion that may preclude resection and may provide enough additional length on the vessels to make resection possible. Going into the pericardium is often the key move in assessing resectability of a central lesion.

Once it has been established that resection is possible and the vessels are encircled (**Fig. 17-2**), the proximal main stem bronchus is dissected. Depending on the location of the tumor, division of the azygos vein may facilitate this dissection as the vein traverses the bronchus just proximal to the takeoff of the right upper lobe (**Fig. 17-3**). This is a consistent landmark. The dissection around the bronchus is carried out with the lung retracted anteriorly. Once the artery has been dissected, it is easy to encircle the bronchus after the pleura overlying the subcarinal space has been incised. Either a finger or a blunt right angle is passed around the right main bronchus.

The location of the tumor dictates to some extent the order in which the vascular structures are divided. With proximal involvement of the artery, it is often easier to divide the veins first, followed by the bronchus, leaving the artery until last when the exposure is at a maximum. I prefer to divide the main pulmonary artery and the superior and inferior pulmonary veins between rows of staples placed by a vascular stapler (**Fig. 17-4**). Alternatively a vessel may be divided between clamps and closed with a running monofilament nonabsorbable suture. In my opinion, it is not adequate to place only a tie on the main pulmonary artery or on the veins; proximal vessels should at least be doubly ligated with a suture ligature if a stapler is not used or the vessels are not sutured. Occasionally, divid-

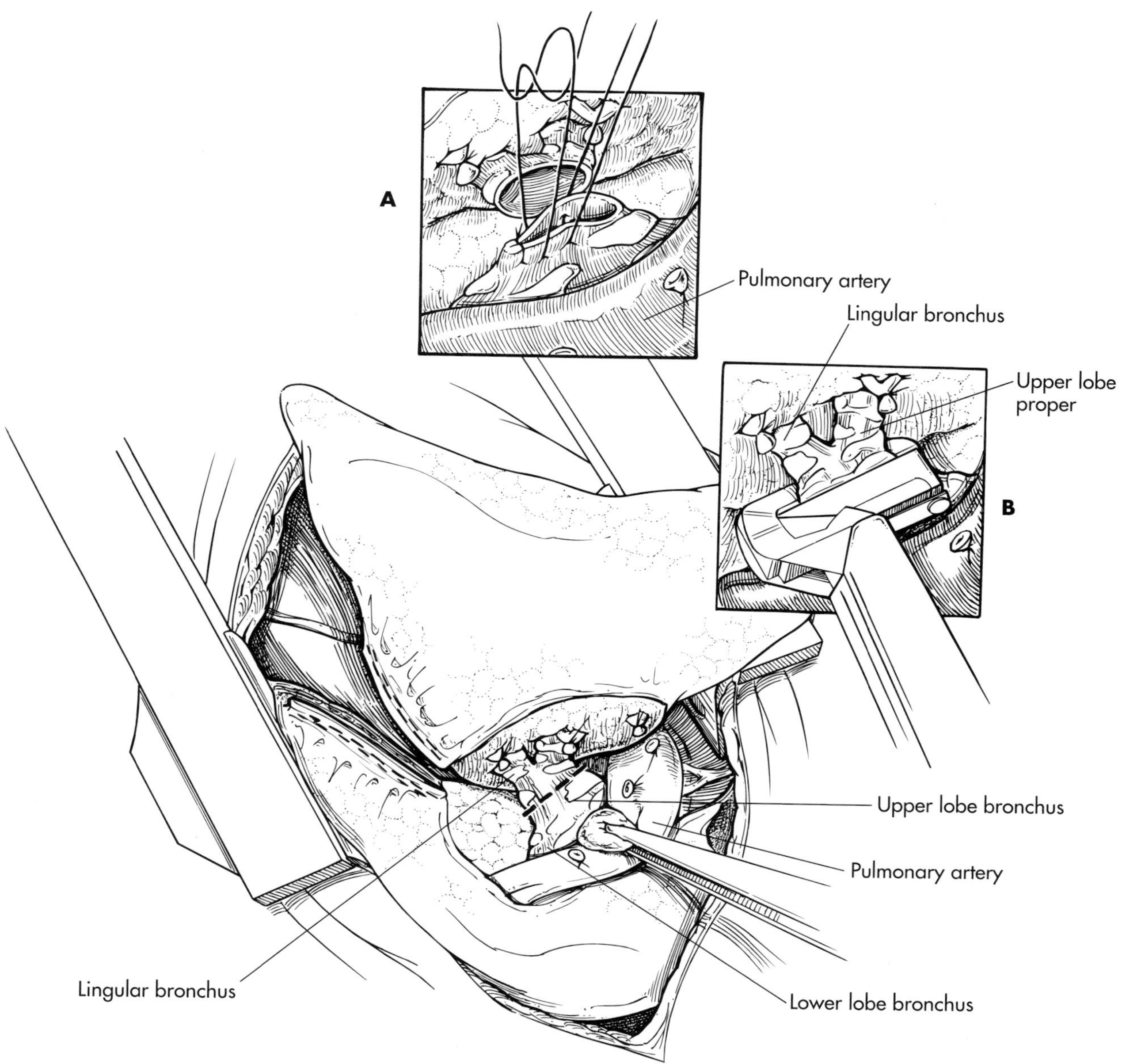
A
Pulmonary artery
Lingular bronchus
Upper lobe proper
B
Upper lobe bronchus
Pulmonary artery
Lingular bronchus
Lower lobe bronchus

FIGURE 18-6

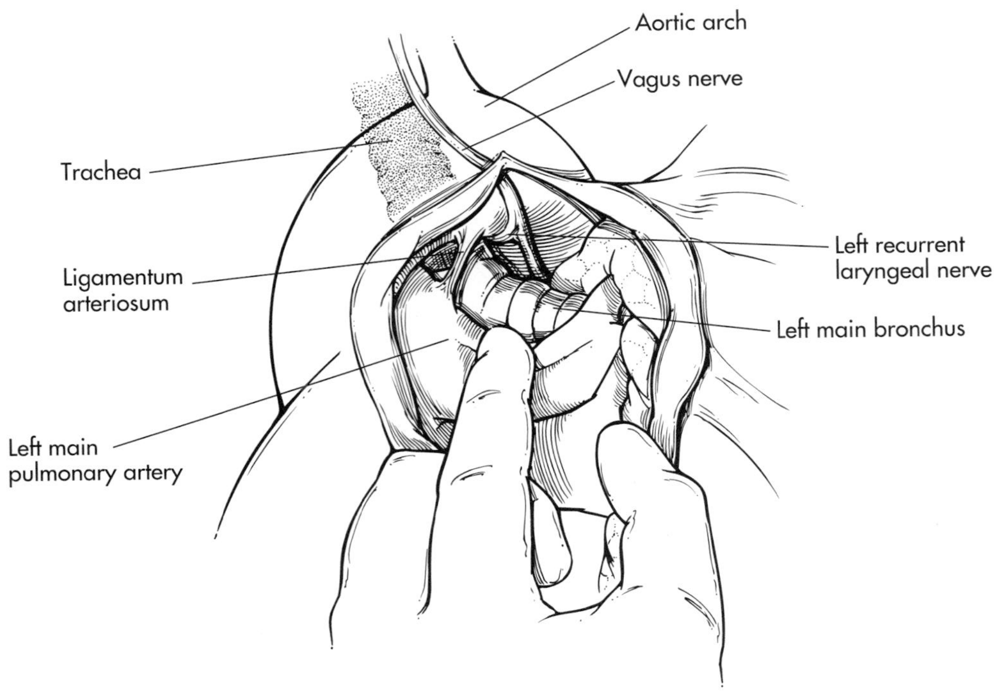

FIGURE 18-7

bronchus. Small vagal branches going to the lung are divided between metal clips. The contents of the subcarinal space are removed using blunt and sharp dissection along with the liberal use of metal clips. The left paratracheal and tracheobronchial angle lymph nodes are most easily sampled at mediastinoscopy, but if exposure of the superior mediastinum is needed, it is obtained by dissecting superiorly along the trachea accessed via the aortopulmonary window (**Fig. 18-7**). Great care must be taken to avoid the left recurrent laryngeal nerve, which "recurs" around the ligamentum arteriosum. If the patient is hoarse in the postoperative period the vocal cords must be examined to assure that the left vocal cord is moving. If the left vocal cord is paralyzed, the patient's ability to cough and clear secretions in the postoperative period will be markedly impaired and aspiration is a potential problem.

Bibliography

Graeber GM, Collins JJH, DeShong JL, et al: Are sutures better than staples for closing bronchi and pulmonary vessels? *Ann Thorac Surg* 51:901-904, 1991.

Patterson GA, Piazza D, Pearson FG, et al: Significance of metastatic disease in subaortic lymph nodes, *Ann Thorac Surg* 43:155-159, 1987.

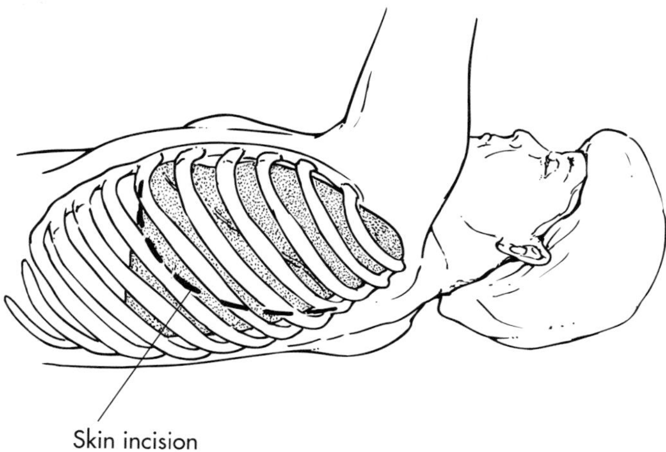

FIGURE 20-1

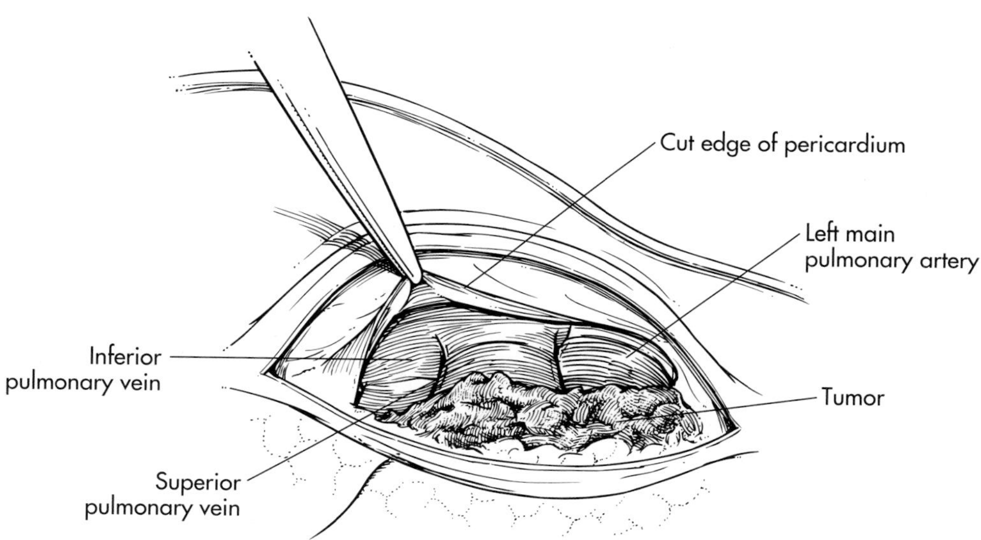

FIGURE 20-2

encasing the hilum, further exploration is required and the pericardium should be incised along the length of the hilum to permit a finger to be inserted (**Fig. 20-2**). This allows assessment of the extent of involvement of the atrium and the confluence of the pulmonary veins as well as proximal involvement of the pulmonary artery. The pericardial incision should be made posterior to the phrenic nerve (on the lung side of the nerve), if possible. Damage to the nerve should be avoided and the nerve sacrificed only if resection is possible and the nerve is involved by tumor. Extensive proximal (medial) invasion of the atrium often precludes resection since one is limited as to how much atrium may be safely and prudently resected. How extensive is too extensive is difficult to judge, but the feasibility of resection is borderline once involvement of the venous confluence is recognized. It is important to assess involvement of the posterior hilum as well, and to ensure resectability, it must be possible to pass a finger around the hilum. Often one encounters a shelf of tumor extending further medially when one palpates the posterior hilum; this precludes safe resection.

The proximal extent of involvement of the pulmonary artery must also be ascertained via intrapericardial exploration. Division of the ligamentum arteriosum allows for a complete assessment

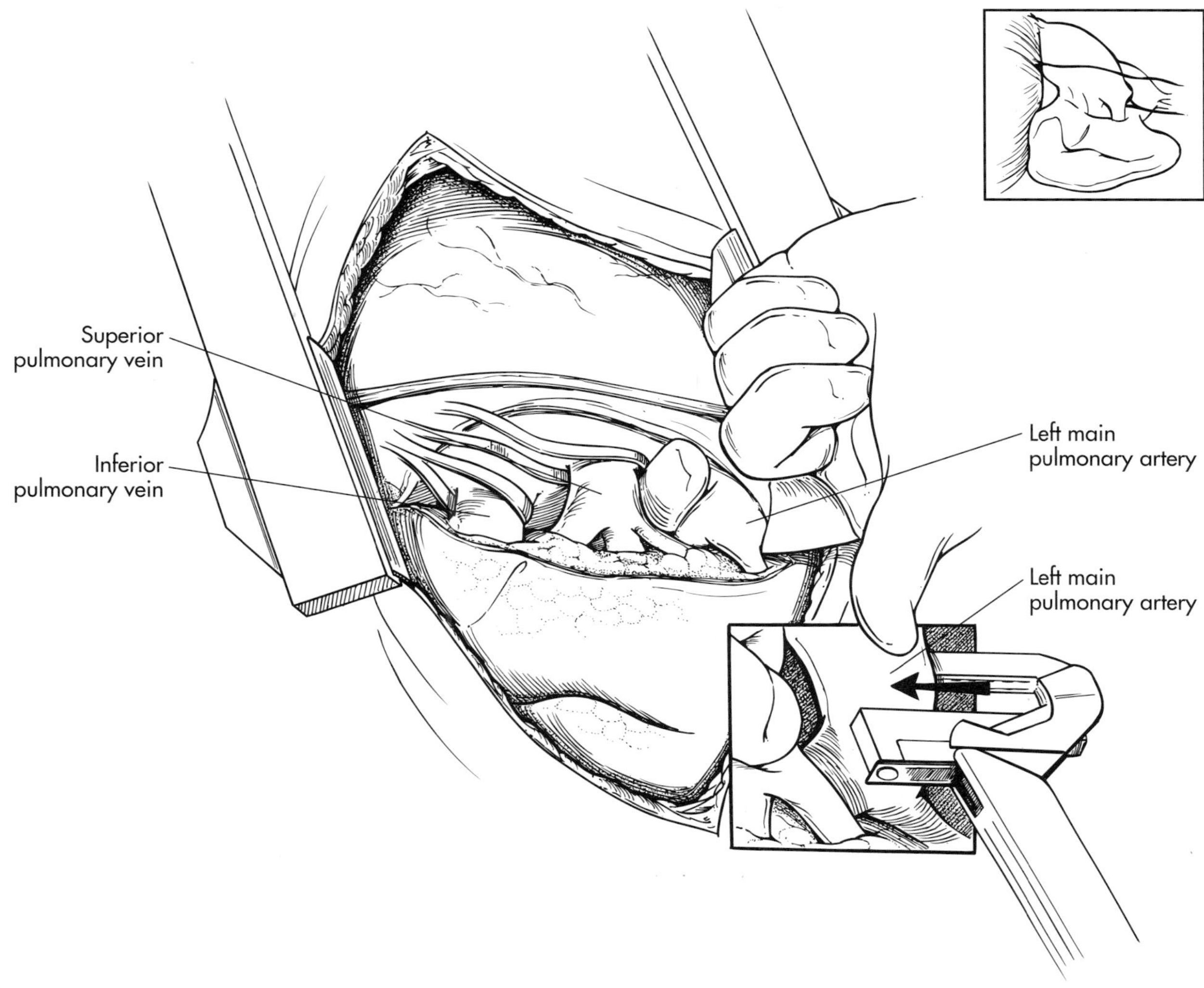

FIGURE 20-3

of the entire length of the left main pulmonary artery and may be necessary to complete a resection. Rarely does involvement of the bronchus determine resectablity, but this should be assessed before "burning any bridges."

Once it has been established that the lesion is resectable and that pneumonectomy is required, the hilar structures must be mobilized. If an intrapericardial assessment has been necessary, the pulmonary artery is encircled within the pericardium, as are the superior and inferior pulmonary veins. If the procedure is feasible, the hilar pleura is incised anteriorly and superiorly with the lung retracted posteriorly (**Fig. 20-3**). The left main pulmonary artery is encircled either with a blunt-tipped clamp or preferably with a finger. The superior pulmonary vein is also encircled and the inferior pulmonary ligament is divided, allowing the inferior pulmonary vein to be encircled. The order in which the hilar structures are divided varies depending on the location of the tumor. Occasionally, it may even be preferable to divide the left main bronchus before dividing any of the vascular structures. I prefer to divide the main pulmonary artery between two rows of vascular staples (**Fig. 20-3, *inset***). Alternatively, a vascular clamp is placed on the proximal pulmonary artery, and the artery is divided and closed with a running monofilament suture. The superior pulmonary vein is also divided between rows of vascular staples or may be clamped and sewn, as previously described (**Fig. 20-4**). The inferior pulmonary vein may be approached from either the anterior or posterior aspect of

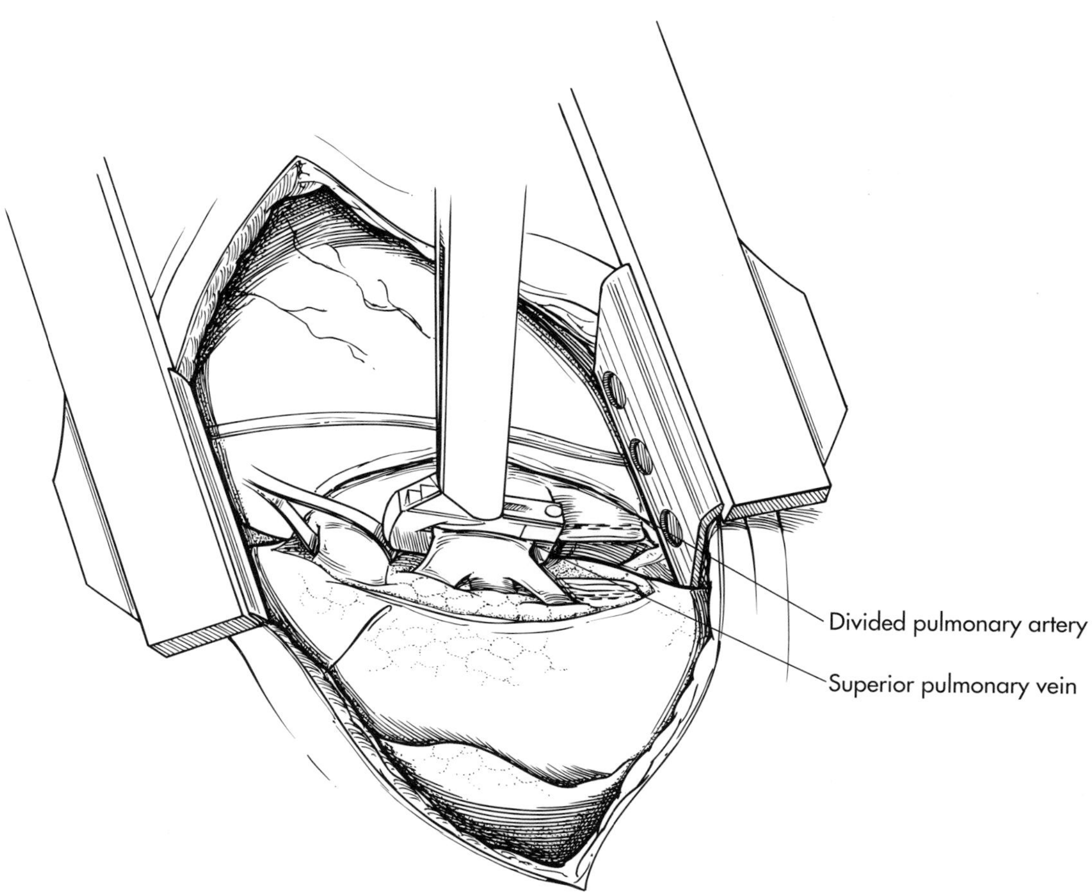

FIGURE 20-4

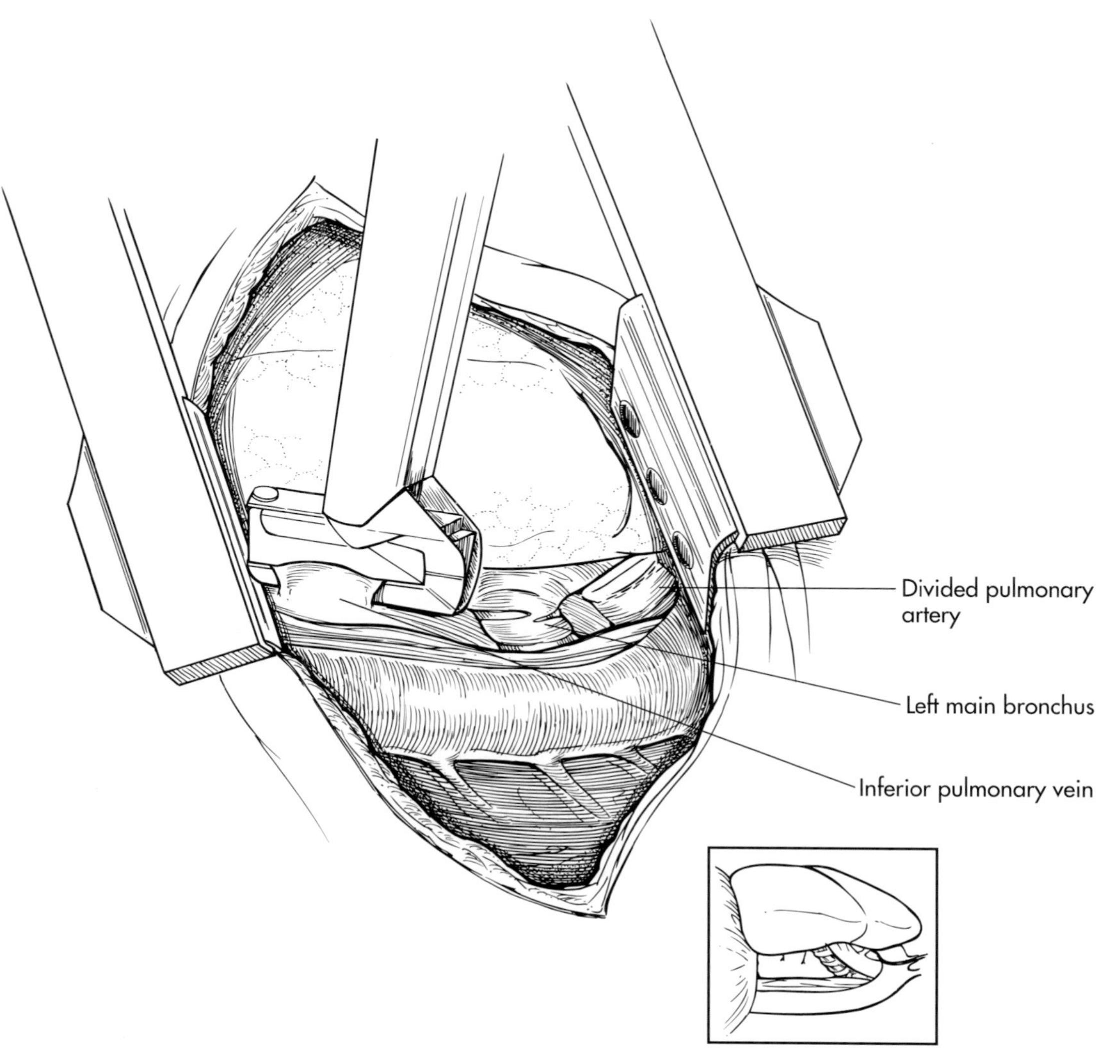

FIGURE 20-5

the hilum, stapled or clamped, and divided (**Fig. 20-5**). The bronchus is approached from the posterior aspect of the hilum with the lung retracted anteriorly and divided as close as possible to the carina (**Fig. 20-6**). Whether a stapler is used (**Fig. 20-6, *inset A***) or the bronchus is cut and sutured is a matter of personal preference. I favor the mechanical stapler as long as there is no involvement close to the origin of the bronchus. I sew a flap of parietal pleura to the bronchial stump using fine silk sutures to reinforce the bronchial closure of a pneumonectomy stump (**Fig. 20-6, *inset B***). This flap is usually based superiorly and takes the pleura overlying the descending thoracic aorta for approximately 5 cm.

If the pericardium has been open, it must be closed to prevent herniation of the heart into the pneumonectomy space. This is important for either a right or left pneumonectomy. If the pericardium only has been incised, a few sutures may be all that is required to close the defect but constriction of the heart must be avoided. If a piece of pericardium has been excised, a patch of prosthetic material should be used to close the defect. The prosthetic patch should be loosely sewn into place to prevent even minimal tamponade physiology.

A chest tube is placed into the pneumonectomy space to allow the position of the mediastinum to equilibrate and to monitor bleeding into the space. The tube is removed within 24 hours.

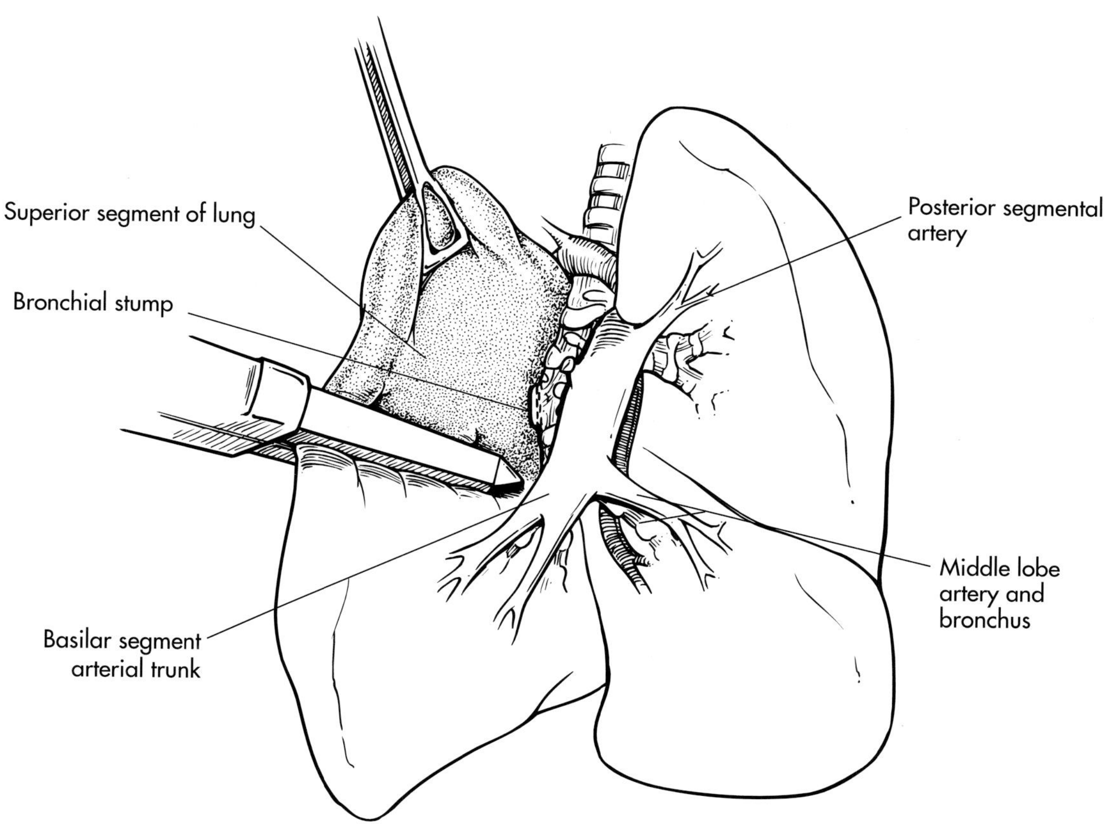
Superior segment of lung
Bronchial stump
Posterior segmental artery
Middle lobe artery and bronchus
Basilar segment arterial trunk

FIGURE 22-6

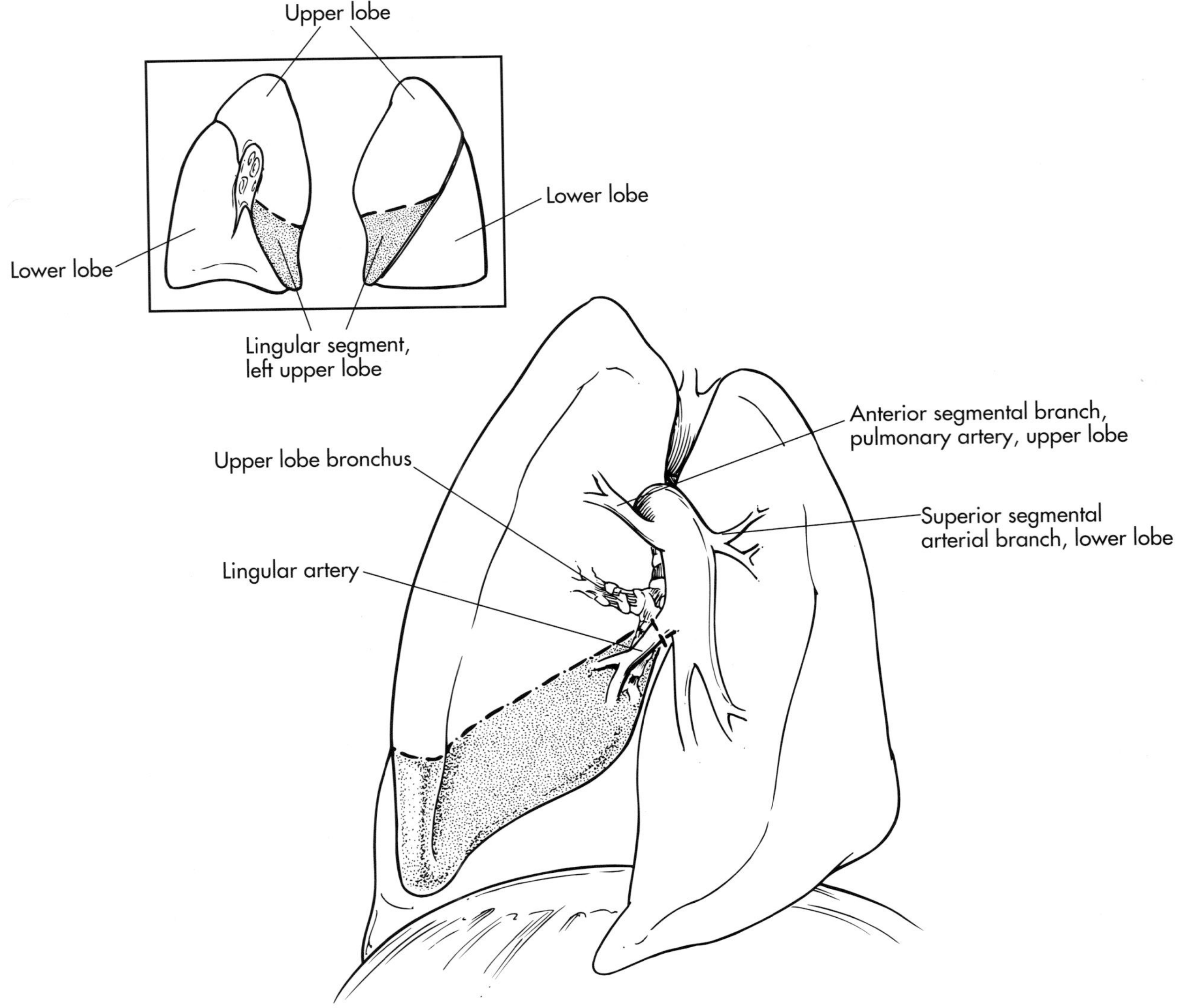

FIGURE 22-7

LINGULAR SEGMENTECTOMY

Lingular segmentectomy is the prototype segmental resection since anatomically the bronchovascular structures are well defined. The chest is entered through a thoracotomy incision, and the chest is inspected to ensure resectability and absence of pleural metastatic disease. An assessment is made as to whether lingular segmentectomy is adequate to encompass the lesion (**Fig. 22-7, *inset***).

If the lobar fissure is well developed, the pleura overlying the pulmonary artery within the fissure is incised and the arterial plane dissected. Within the fissure the anterior segmental branch of the artery is first encountered on the superior aspect of the artery, while slightly inferior and on the inferior aspect of the artery lies the branch to the superior segment of the lower lobe. Following the artery further distally the lingular branch or branches are seen (**Fig. 22-7**). Often there is more than one lingular branch, and these are ligated and divided.

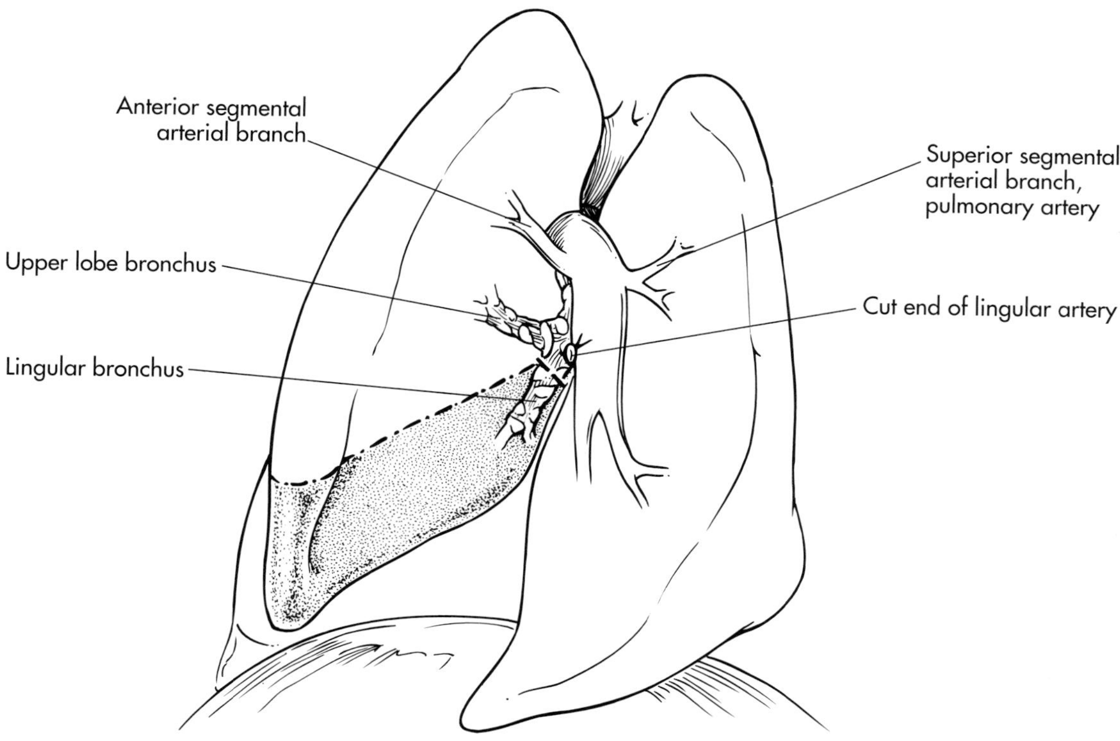

FIGURE 22-8

Once the arterial branch is divided, the lingular bronchus is found slightly inferior and posterior (deep) (**Fig. 22-8**). It is usually safest to identify the bifurcation between the lingular bronchus and the upper lobe bronchus before dividing. Once a positive identification of the lingular bronchus is made, the bronchus is skeletonized, encircled, stapled, and divided. Alternatively, the bronchus may be divided and sewn closed with interrupted sutures of absorbable material.

There is a discrete lingular venous branch that drains into the superior pulmonary vein and is identified with the lung retracted posteriorly by incising the hilar pleura overlying the vein (**Fig. 22-9**). The lingular vein is ligated and divided. After the complete division of the bronchovascular structures to the lingula, the line of division of the parenchyma is usually evident. The anterior portion of the oblique fissure is completed with a firing of the linear stapler placed in a plane developed just superior to the artery and distal to the divided lingular arterial branch. The division of the parenchyma between the lingula and the upper lobe proper is also accomplished with a linear stapler; the stapler placement is guided by the location of the bronchial stump.

Mediastinal lymph nodes, especially in the aortopulmonary window, should be taken for staging purposes. The chest is closed in the usual fashion after the placement of chest tubes.

Other segmental resections are merely variations on what has been described previously. As mentioned, the key to segmental resection is identification of the segmental artery. Especially with upper lobe lesions, it may be somewhat difficult to identify the segmental artery supplying the segment of interest. It is probably best to secure proximal control of the main pulmonary artery before beginning the dissection of a segmental arterial branch.

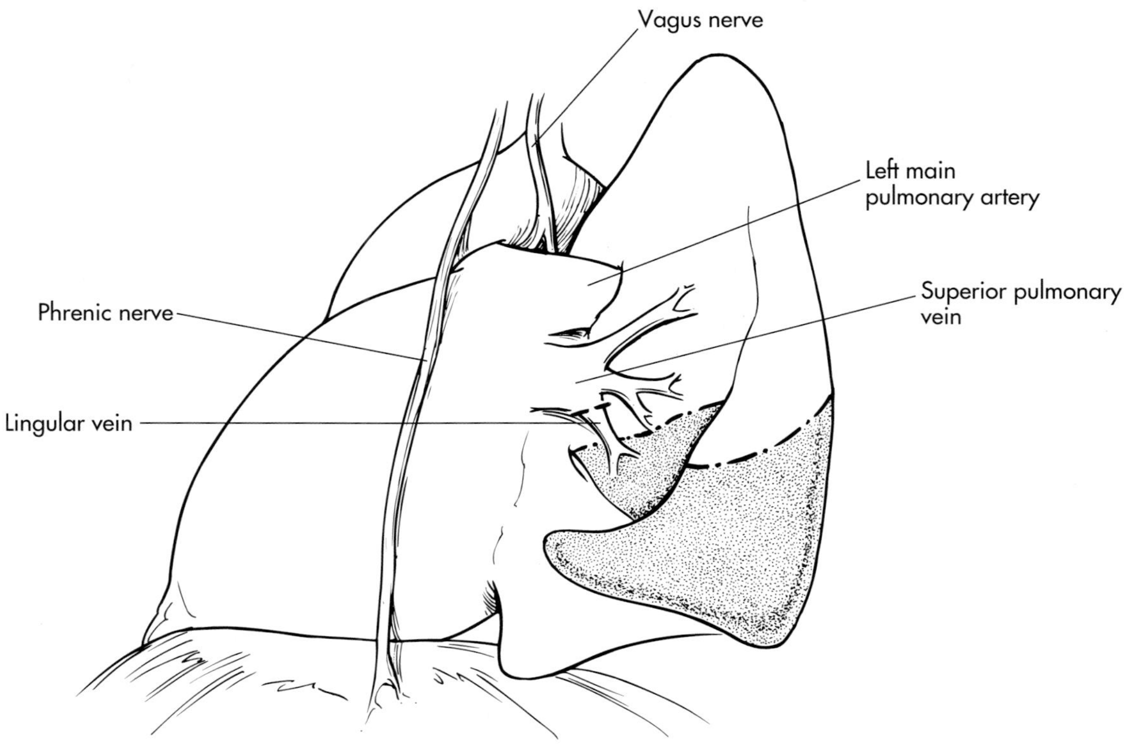

FIGURE 22-9

Bibliography

Churchill ED and Belsey R: Segmental pneumonectomy in bronchiectasis: the lingula segment of the left upper lobe, *Ann Surg* 109:481–499, 1939.

Miller JI and Hatcher CR: Limited resection of bronchogenic carcinoma in the patient with marked impairment of pulmonary function, *Ann Thorac Surg* 44:340–343, 1987.

Warren WH and Faber LP: Segmentectomy versus lobectomy in patients with stage I pulmonary carcinoma: five-year survival and patterns of intrathoracic recurrence, *J Thorac Cardiovasc Surg* 107:1087–1093, 1994.

CHAPTER 25

Wedge Excision of Pulmonary Nodule

The standard resection for a malignant lung lesion remains anatomic resection, most commonly lobectomy. There are some circumstances—compromised pulmonary function and metastasectomy for multiple lesions to name two—where wedge excision is not only acceptable but preferable. When operating for a solitary pulmonary nodule where a preoperative diagnosis has not been established, wedge excision is the usual first step. Once the diagnosis has been established, a decision regarding further resection is made. Usually, in these situations, we perform this initial exploration and wedge excision via a videothoracoscopic technique.

As illustrated here, the area of lung to be excised is grasped with a lung clamp and a row of staples is placed using a linear stapler (**Fig. 25-1**). The staple line should be placed far enough away to obtain a clear margin. A second firing of the stapler, as shown, completes the wedge excision of the nodule and the surrounding normal parenchyma. This procedure is simple when the nodule is located on the periphery of lung. When the nodule is deeper and on a "flat" surface of the lung, a wedge excision can be extremely difficult since there is no "edge." For nodules in a difficult location, at times the nodule may be grasped and lifted upward and the stapler fired beneath it. At other times, the only alternative is a direct precision cautery excision where a cylinder of parenchyma surrounding the nodule is removed along with the lesion. Care should be taken to clip vessels and bronchi as they are encountered. Surprisingly, the air leak following this excision usually stops very quickly and rarely presents a problem.

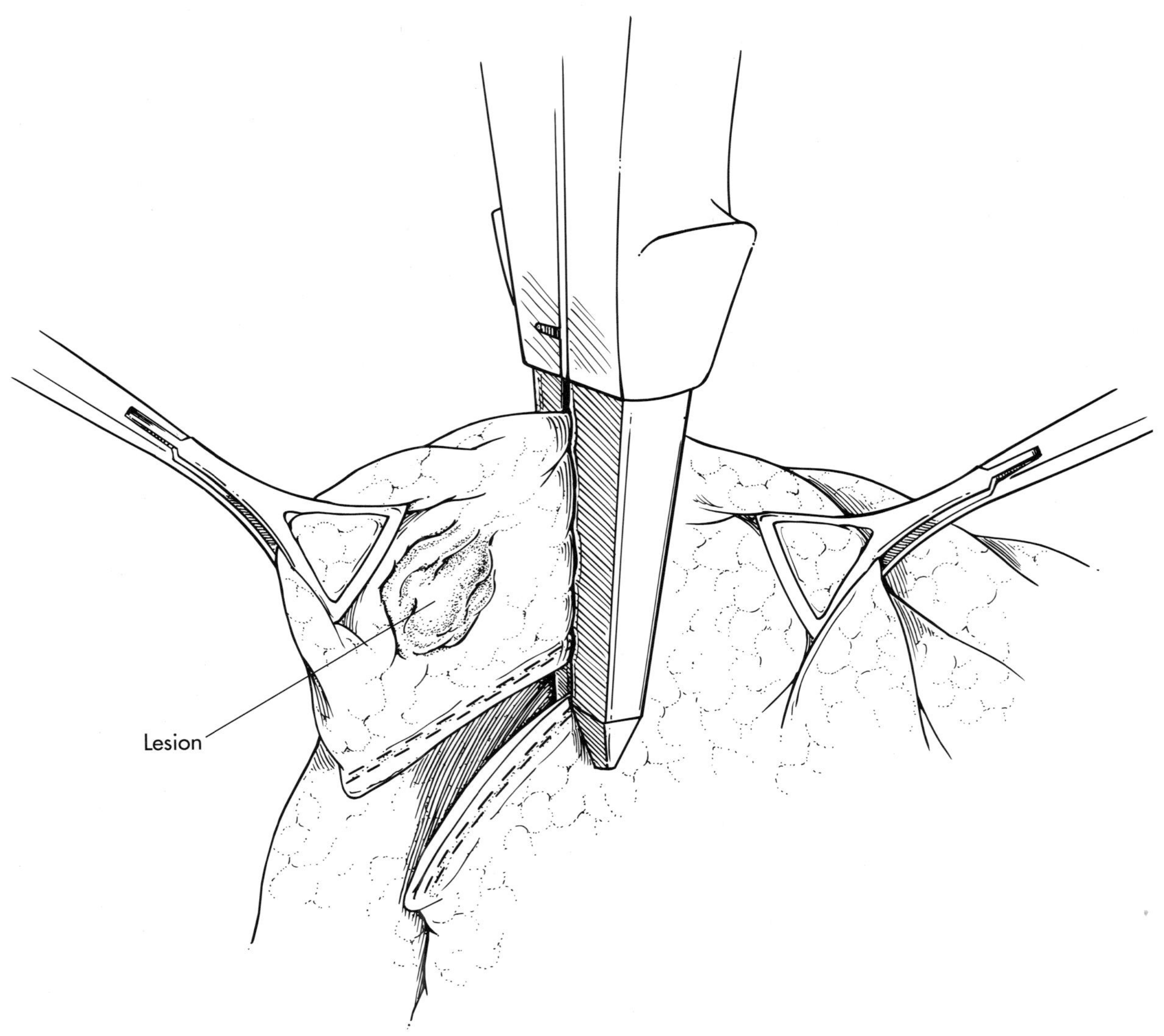

FIGURE 25-1

Bibliography

Errett LE, Wilson J, Chiu RC, et al: Wedge resection as an alternate procedure for peripheral bronchogenic carcinoma in poor risk patients, *J Thorac Cardiovasc Surg* 90:656–661, 1985.

Velasco FT, Rusch VW, and Ginsberg RJ: Thoracoscopic management of chest neoplasms, *Semin Laparoscopic Surg* 1:43–51, 1994.

PART V

Chest Wall Procedures

CHAPTER 26

Transaxillary First Rib Resection

The diagnosis of thoracic outlet syndrome, a nerve entrapment and only rarely a vascular compression syndrome, is difficult because there are no objective criteria or studies on which the diagnosis may be based. Usually it is a diagnosis of exclusion, with the exception of the occasional patient who presents with a cervical rib or the rare patient with effort-induced thrombosis of the subclavian vein (Paget-Schroetter syndrome). There are no typical radiologic or physical examination findings, but cervical disk and carpal tunnel syndrome should be ruled out. Often, the patient presents with a history of upper extremity or shoulder trauma, after which they note the onset of pain. The type of pain, severity, and distribution vary widely, and there is no typical pattern. Patients should be encouraged to pursue all nonoperative means, usually a physical therapy regimen, before any consideration of operation. When a well-constructed physical therapy program provides little or no relief, in selected patients, decompression of the thoracic outlet by resection of the first rib relieves symptoms for some. The long-term follow-up of these patients indicates that some develop recurrent symptoms over a period of years. Again, with no objective measurements it is difficult to assess the contribution, if any, that first rib resection makes in the management of this syndrome. Indeed, many knowledgeable physicians have questioned even the existence of this so-called syndrome, which further calls the operation into question.

Recognizing the controversy, I present details of the operation mainly because it should be performed only occasionally and thus there should be a source where the important details of the procedure are available for review. Resection of the first rib may be performed via a supraclavicular approach, a high posterior thoracotomy, or a transaxillary approach. The supraclavicular approach requires dissection in an area rich with important structures such as the subclavian vessels and the brachial plexus just to reach the first rib. For those surgeons intimately familiar with the anatomy of the supraclavicular region, this approach may prove to be the one of choice. The posterior thoracotomy required to expose the first rib is an extensive destructive procedure that requires division of the trapezius muscle, the latissimus dorsi muscle, and the serratus anterior muscle and elevation of the scapula off the chest wall. This is the preferred approach for a secondary procedure to remove a remnant of the first rib that has been left after an initial procedure. I prefer, as do most thoracic surgeons performing this procedure, the transaxillary approach, which is the most direct and least destructive.

DESCRIPTION OF THE PROCEDURE

The patient is placed on the table in the lateral decubitus position. The ipsilateral arm, axilla, and chest are prepared and draped with the arm placed in a stockinette so that it may be manipulated as the exposure demands. The second assistant holds the arm, resting it on his or her own arm (**Fig. 26-1**). The arm is abducted to expose the axilla, and a skin incision is made inferior to the hair line. The

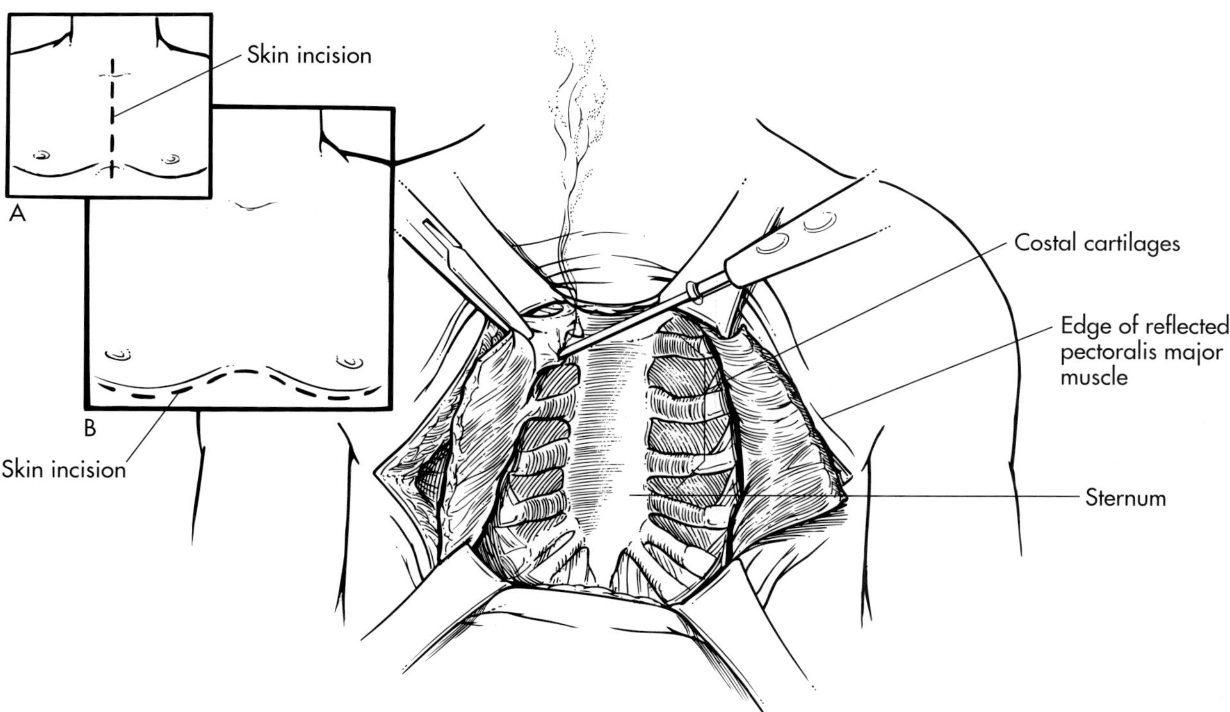
Skin incision
A
B
Skin incision
Costal cartilages
Edge of reflected pectoralis major muscle
Sternum

FIGURE 27-1

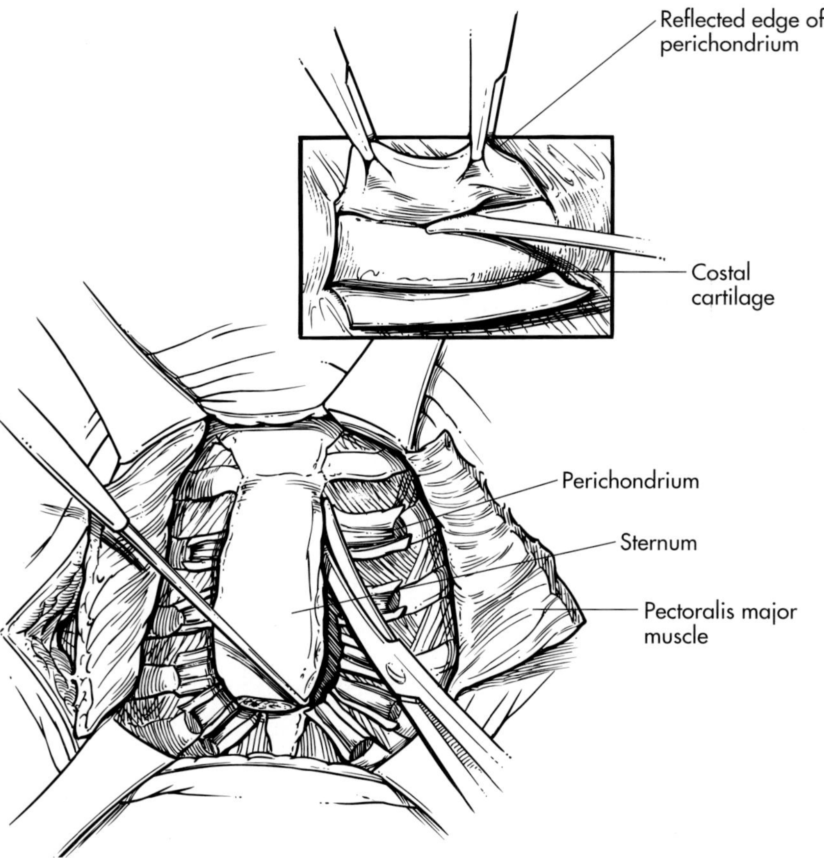
Reflected edge of perichondrium
Costal cartilage
Perichondrium
Sternum
Pectoralis major muscle

FIGURE 27-2

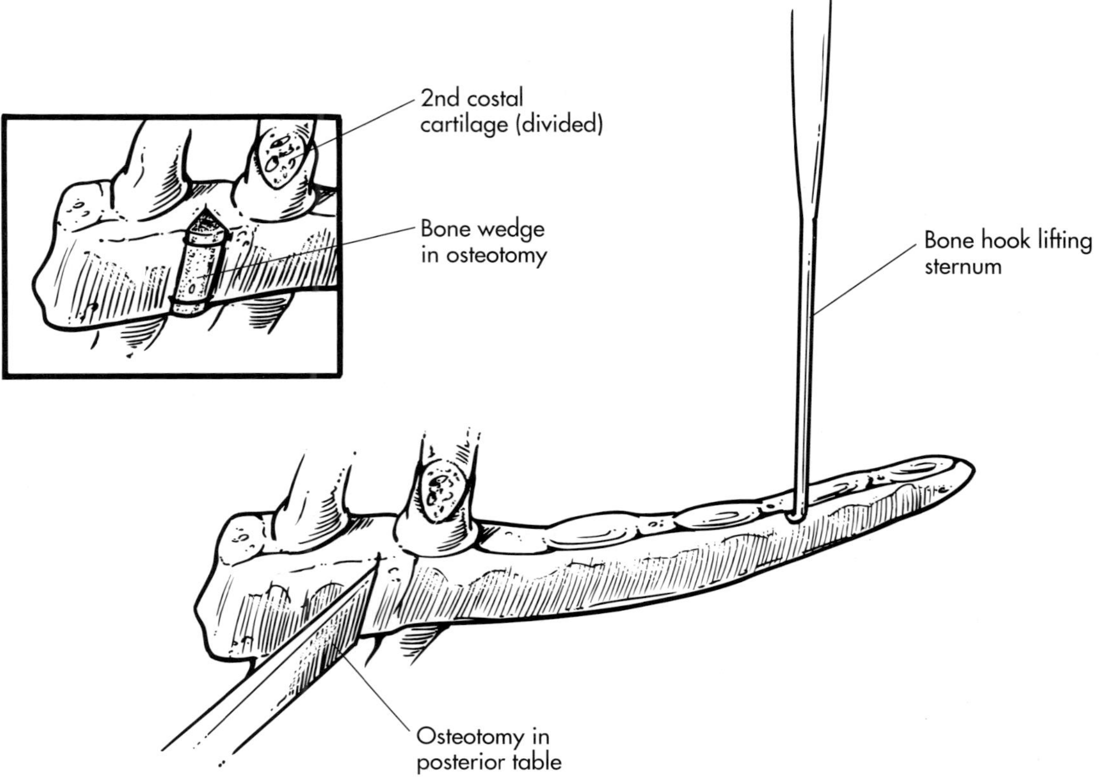

FIGURE 27-3

forcibly pulled anteriorly to fracture, but not separate, the anterior table (**Fig. 27-3**). This completes the total mobilization of the sternum. A piece of rib of a size to fit within the osteotomy is harvested and wedged into position to keep the sternum pitched anteriorly (**Fig. 27-3, *inset***). Two to three wires are placed through the manubrium around the bone wedge and back up through the body of the sternum to secure the bone wedge in position. This can be a difficult move to accomplish, and one must be sure that the wires are in the correct position and twisted tightly enough to maintain the bone wedge in place. This is the main stabilization for the repair aided by another point of fixation created by the overriding second costal cartilage, which is stabilized with either a heavy silk suture or wire (**Fig. 27-4, *inset***).

A third point of fixation may be achieved by placing a fixation wire (Kirschner) through the sternum and securing the wire to rib on either side with another wire placed through the rib (**Fig. 27-4**). The Kirschner wire should be of a gauge that allows it to be bent to an appropriate shape to maintain the sternum in the position of fixation directed anteriorly. This degree of fixation should provide a margin of safety in the postoperative period until healing occurs.

An occasional accompaniment to the cartilage deformity that defines pectus excavatum is a rotational defect of the bony sternum itself. This sternal defect is always a rotation toward the right and must be corrected at the time of the cartilaginous excision. It is important to point out the wide spectrum of pathology that may be encountered when dealing with pectus excavatum and to stress that the surgeon must be somewhat creative to achieve the best results. It is impossible in a discussion such as this to even begin to catalog all the possible variations and degrees of the pectus deformity, but an appreciation of the pathology and a thorough understanding of the fundamental repair allow the surgeon to solve a problem as it is encountered. To correct the rotational deformity, a full-thickness osteotomy is made through the right side of the sternum at the level of the rotation (**Fig. 27-5**). On the left side of the sternum opposite the full-thickness osteotomy, a second cut is made through

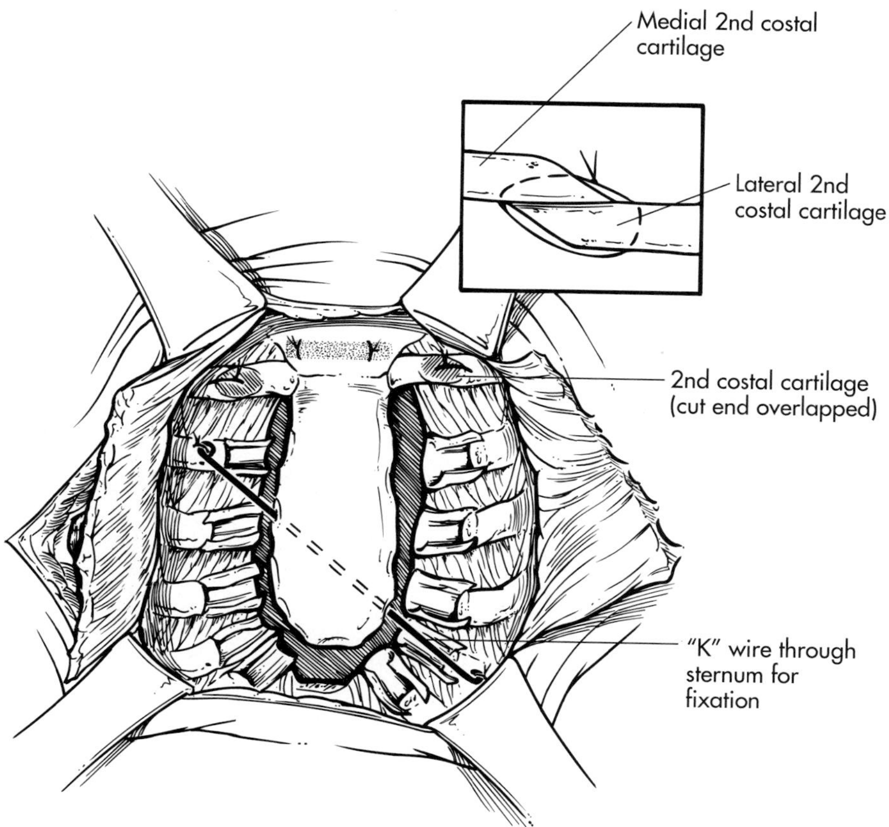
Medial 2nd costal cartilage
Lateral 2nd costal cartilage
2nd costal cartilage (cut end overlapped)
"K" wire through sternum for fixation

FIGURE 27-4

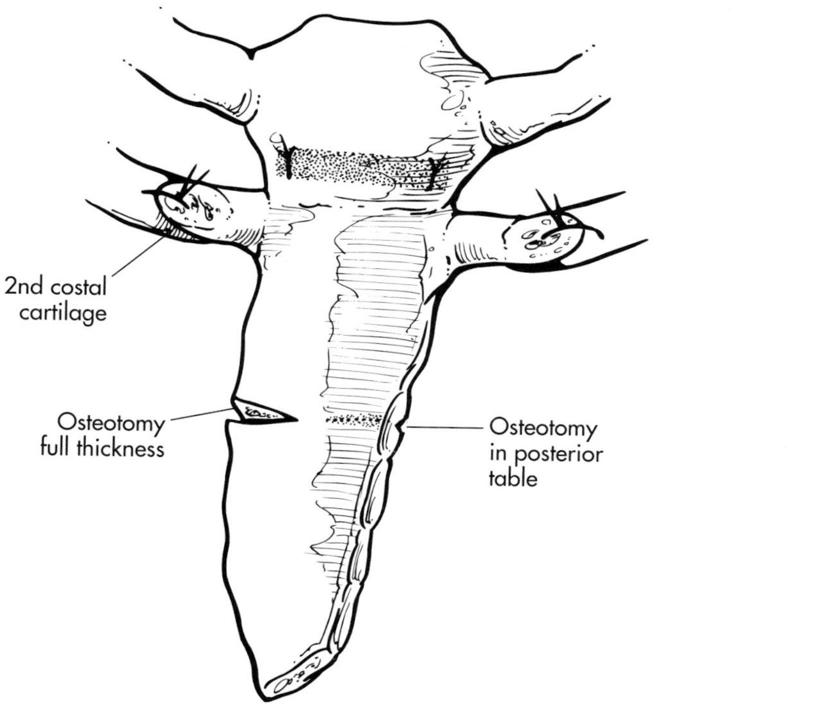
2nd costal cartilage
Osteotomy full thickness
Osteotomy in posterior table

FIGURE 27-5

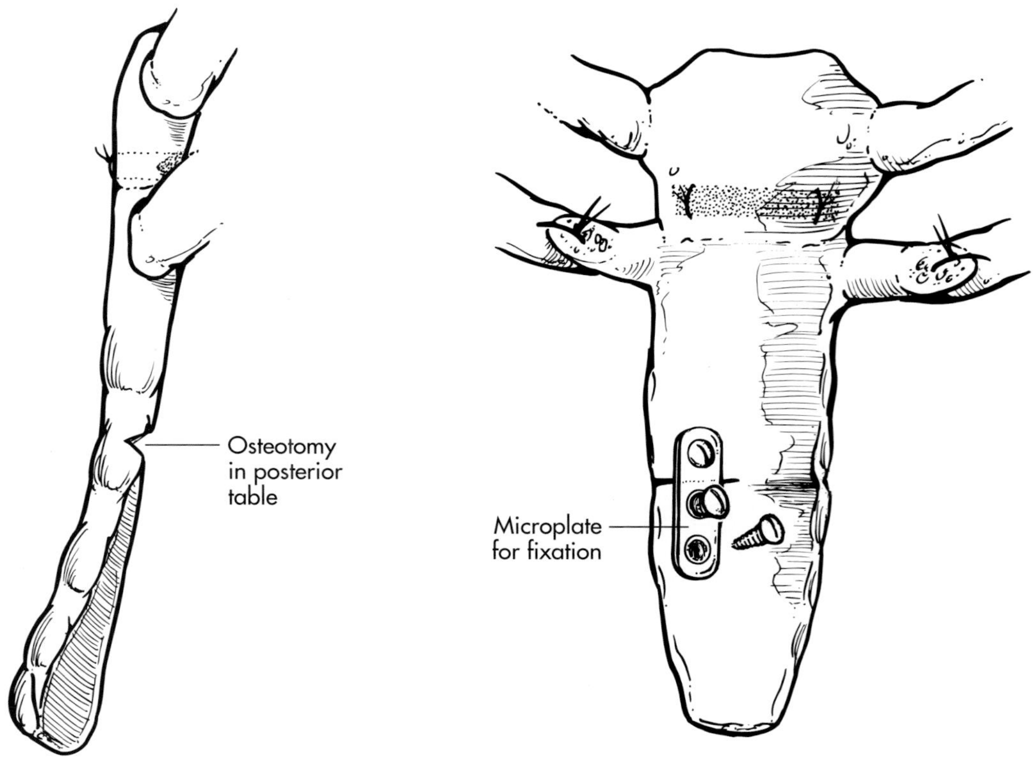

FIGURE 27-6 **FIGURE 27-7**

the posterior table of the sternum, allowing the bone to be rotated into a normal orientation (**Fig. 27-6**). The correction of the rotation is fixed in place using microplates and screws (AO system), with the surgeon having bent the plates appropriately to maintain the correction (**Fig. 27-7**). Using microplates and screws, in our opinion, represents a significant improvement over the use of wire to maintain the derotation.

The pectoralis muscles are reapproximated in the midline overlying the sternum. The subcutaneous tissue is closed. Suction drains should be left in place under the skin flaps if an inframammary incision has been used. The skin is closed with a subcuticular skin suture.

Other variations of the pectus deformity may include the cartilaginous deformity isolated to one side, a mix of unilateral cartilaginous deformity and rotational defect of the sternum, or any number of other combinations. These deformities often present a significant challenge to the surgeon but are better dealt with during the primary procedure than counting on a secondary procedure to "complete" the repair.

Bibliography

Golladay ES and Wagner CW: Pectus excavatum: a 15-year perspective, *South Med J* 84:1099–1102, 1991.

Haller JA Jr, Scherer LR, Turner CS, et al: Evolving management of pectus excavatum based on a single institutional experience of 664 patients, *Ann Surg* 209:578–582, 1989.

Kaguraoka H, Ohnuki T, Itaoka T, et al: Degree of severity of pectus excavatum and pulmonary function in preoperative and postoperative periods, *J Thorac Cardiovasc Surg* 104:1483–1488, 1992.

CHAPTER 28

Chest Wall Resection

Resection of the chest wall is required if a primary lung cancer invades the chest wall, a situation that occurs in approximately 5% of resectable lung cancers. Often, the diagnosis of chest wall invasion is suspected because the patient presents with pain referable to the area where the tumor is located. This is a more reliable predictor of chest wall involvement than either magnetic resonance imaging (MRI) or computed tomographic (CT) scanning, which have limitations in distinguishing abutment from invasion. Direct invasion of the chest wall by a primary lung tumor is not a contraindication to resection, though this belief persists among many of our medical colleagues. With a suspicion of chest wall involvement, however, it becomes even more important to document the status of the mediastinal lymph nodes, since the combination of N2 (mediastinal nodal involvement) and T3 disease (chest wall involvement) is associated with a very poor long-term outlook (0%, 3-year survival). Therefore, I strongly recommend performing mediastinoscopy in these patients even if the CT scan of the chest shows mediastinal lymph nodes that are less than 1.5 cm in size.

Chest wall resection may also be done for primary tumors of the chest wall, though these are, comparatively speaking, quite rare. When they do occur the majority are sarcomas and require a wide resection of chest wall. Benign tumors of rib usually require only resection of the involved rib and perhaps the adjacent rib and rarely require reconstruction. Sternal tumors, essentially all chondrosarcomas, are a separate topic and are not discussed here.

DESCRIPTION OF THE PROCEDURE

The patient is placed in the lateral decubitus position as for a routine thoracotomy (**Fig. 28-1**). If the tumor involves the anterior chest wall, the procedure may be more easily accomplished if the patient is placed in the supine position. Where chest wall involvement is suspected, a muscle-sparing incision should not be used since the ability to travel some distance under the incision is necessary to resect the involved chest wall. For a primary lung tumor the standard posterolateral incision is made except for anterior lesions, for which an inframammary and perhaps a parasternal incision is made. The incision is carried down to the chest wall, dividing the latissimus dorsi and serratus anterior muscles. Unless the tumor is visible coming through the chest wall, it is necessary to enter the chest to assess the extent of chest wall involvement. Usually I enter the chest through the 5th intercostal space, taking care to stay away from the site where the tumor may be present.

Once inside the pleural space it is important to thoroughly explore the chest to rule out diffuse pleural studding with tumor and to palpate the hilum and mediastinum to be sure that resection is feasible. It would be a disaster to complete the chest wall resection only to find that the pulmonary resection is not possible for whatever reason. Once resectability of the lung is assured, the chest wall involvement is assessed. At times, despite the preoperative suspicion, the lesion is found not even to be adherent to the chest wall. Depending on the findings it may be reasonable to develop an

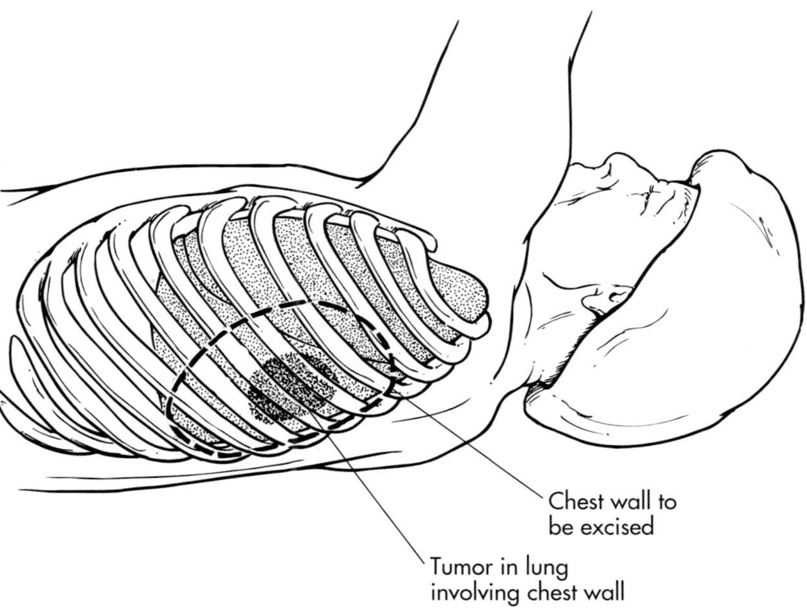

FIGURE 28-1

extrapleural plane of dissection, as sometimes this is all that is required to successfully complete the resection. If there is any question of parietal pleural invasion, then I proceed with chest wall resection. An extrapleural resection alone in the face of parietal pleural invasion is a setup for local recurrence and should be avoided. In most cases, there is little additional morbidity from proceeding with chest wall resection.

Once the decision is made to proceed with chest wall resection, the extent of the resection must be defined. At least one and preferably two ribs above and below the lesion should be included in the resection to minimize the risk of local recurrence. The resection is begun anteriorly by taking a 1- to 2-cm piece of rib at each level. The periosteum is incised, and a piece of rib (approximately 2 cm) is taken after the periosteum is stripped (**Fig. 28-2**). Taking a piece of rib allows for easier identification and ligation of the intercostal bundle as well as provides better access for retraction of the chest wall block. Each piece of rib is submitted separately as the anterior resection margin at each level. The anterior portion of the resection is completed before the posterior aspect of the resection is begun. What is required at the posterior aspect of the resection depends on how far posterior the lesion extends. If rib only has to be taken, the rib is encircled in a subperiosteal plane and cut, after which the intercostal bundle is ligated and divided (**Fig. 28-3**).

At times it may be necessary to disarticulate the rib from the transverse process and the vertebral body. This is accomplished by reflecting the erector spinae ligament to expose the rib at the level of the transverse process. There is a cartilaginous attachment between the neck of the rib and the transverse process that must be incised with electrocautery (**Fig. 28-4**). Once the correct location is found, this cartilaginous attachment melts away as the electrocautery is applied. An osteotome is then inserted between the rib and the transverse process, and force is applied in an anterior direction (**Fig. 28-4, *inset***). This separates the rib from the transverse process and the vertebral body. This maneuver is made easier if the parietal pleura overlying the head of the rib is incised where the rib joins the vertebral body. As the rib is disarticulated from the transverse process and vertebral body, the intercostal nerve must be identified, ligated, and divided as it exits from the neural foramen. Avulsing a nerve root may result in a cerebrospinal fluid leak since the length of the dural sheath on the nerve root is variable.

Once the posterior margin of the resection is complete, the pleura is incised at the inferior and superior margins and the chest wall is fully mobile with the lobe attached. Through the chest wall

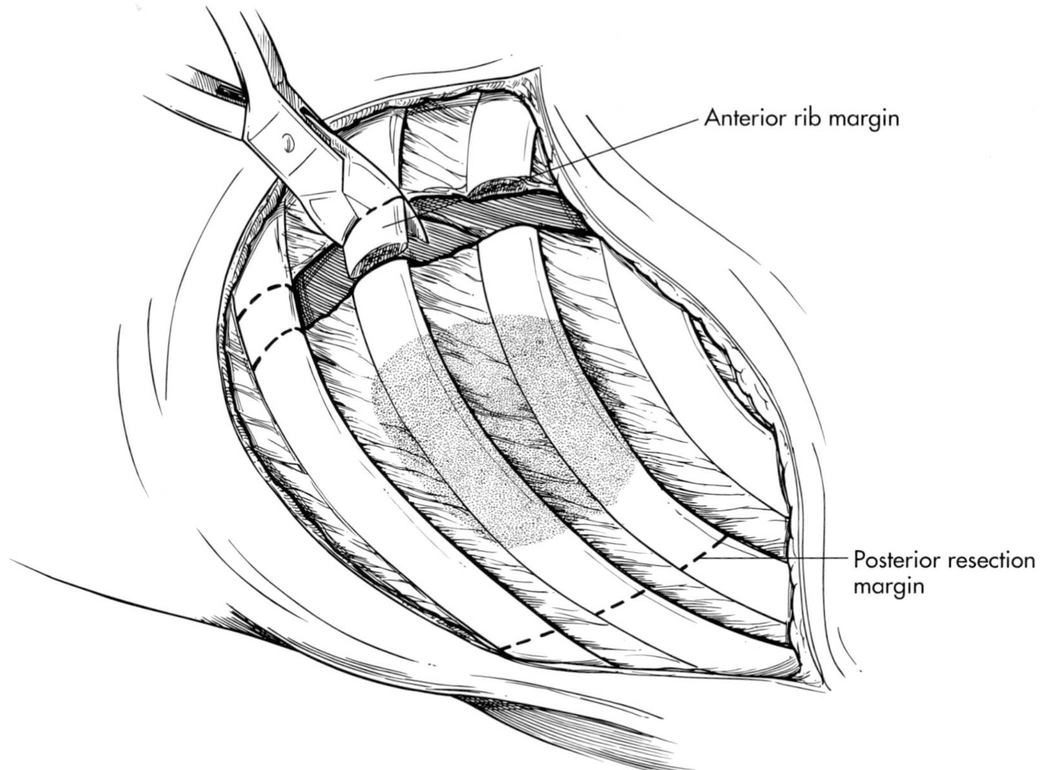

FIGURE 28-2

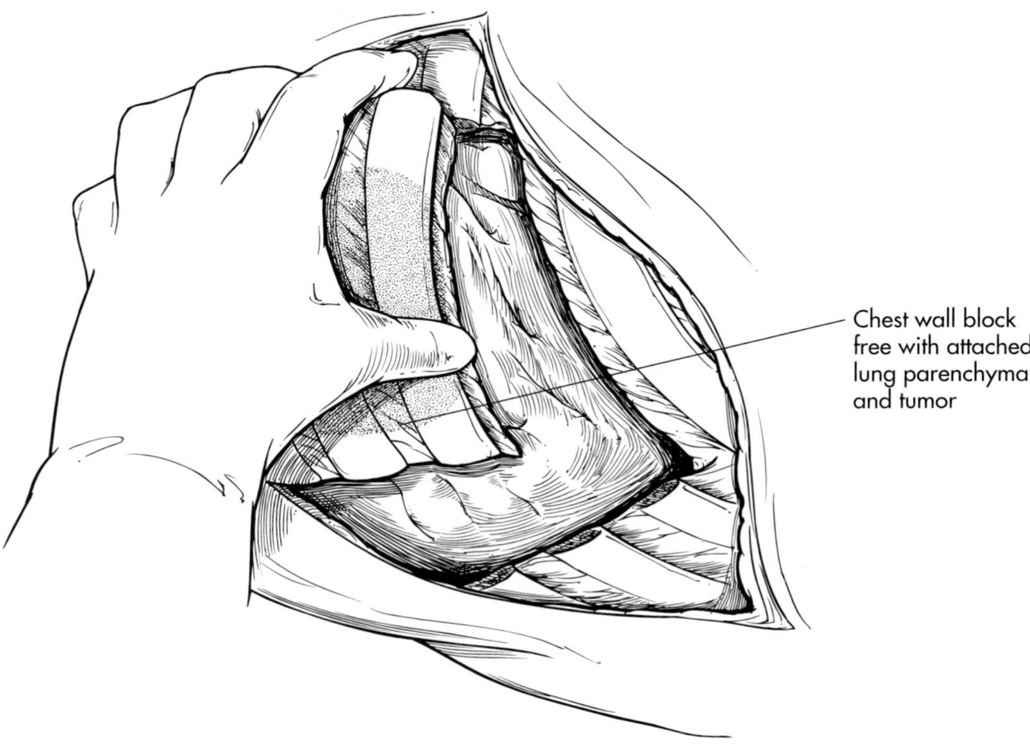

FIGURE 28-3

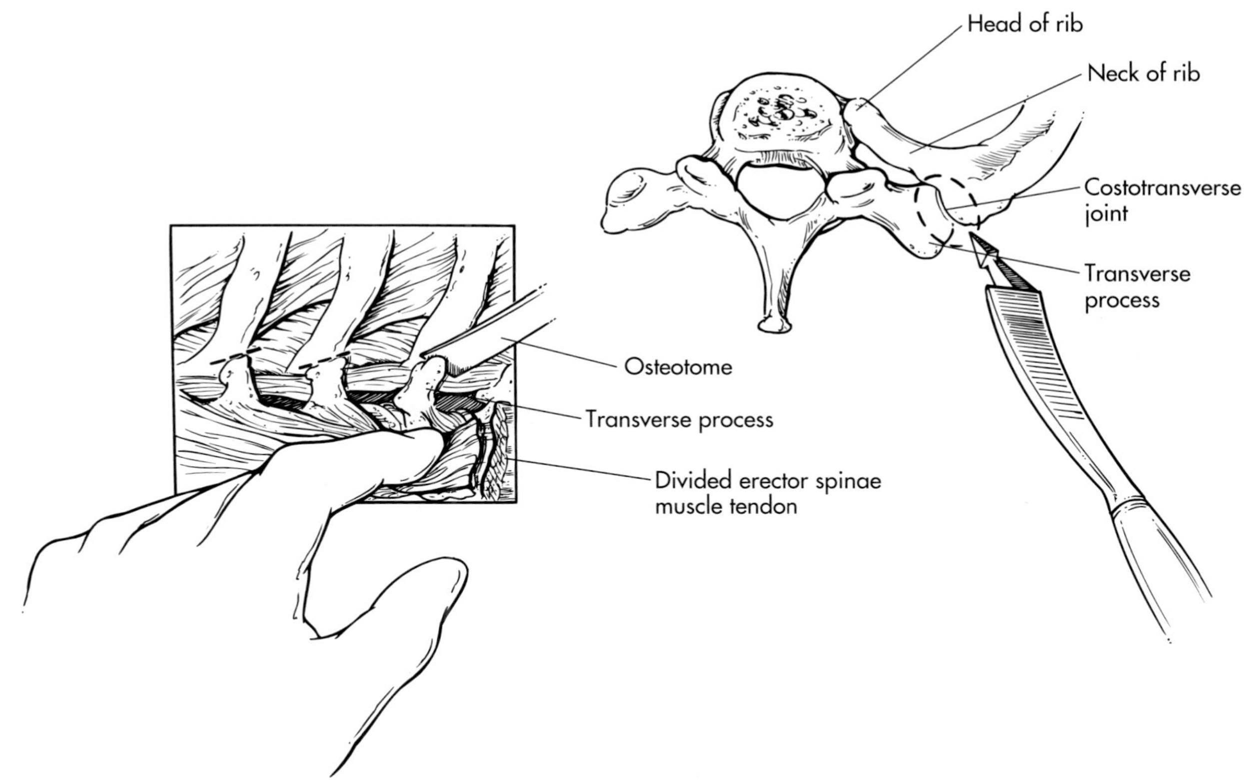

FIGURE 28-4

defect the appropriate lobectomy is performed in the standard fashion (**Fig. 28-5**). This should be accompanied by a mediastinal lymph node dissection. After completion of the lobectomy, chest tubes are placed and a decision made as to whether chest wall reconstruction is required and if so what type of reconstruction.

The resected specimen should be labeled so that the pathologist can accurately report on the margins of resection. The anterior margins are submitted separately as the "plugs" of anterior rib removed. A marking suture should be placed on two additional aspects of the resected specimen to orient the pathologist. It is often a good idea to hand-carry the specimen to the pathologist to demonstrate the margins as marked. If there is any question as to gross disease close to a margin, additional chest wall should be resected. This is particularly difficult, if not impossible, if the posterior margin near vertebral body is questionable, but we readily involve our neurosurgical colleagues and ask that they resect a portion of vertebral body if required. Local recurrence in this area is a particularly difficult problem that results in significant morbidity from pain.

For reconstruction of anterior defects, a prosthetic patch composed of methyl methacrylate cement sandwiched between two sheets of polypropylene mesh and contoured to approximate the curve of the chest wall is used (**Fig. 28-6, *inset***). Depending on the location of a posterior defect, a

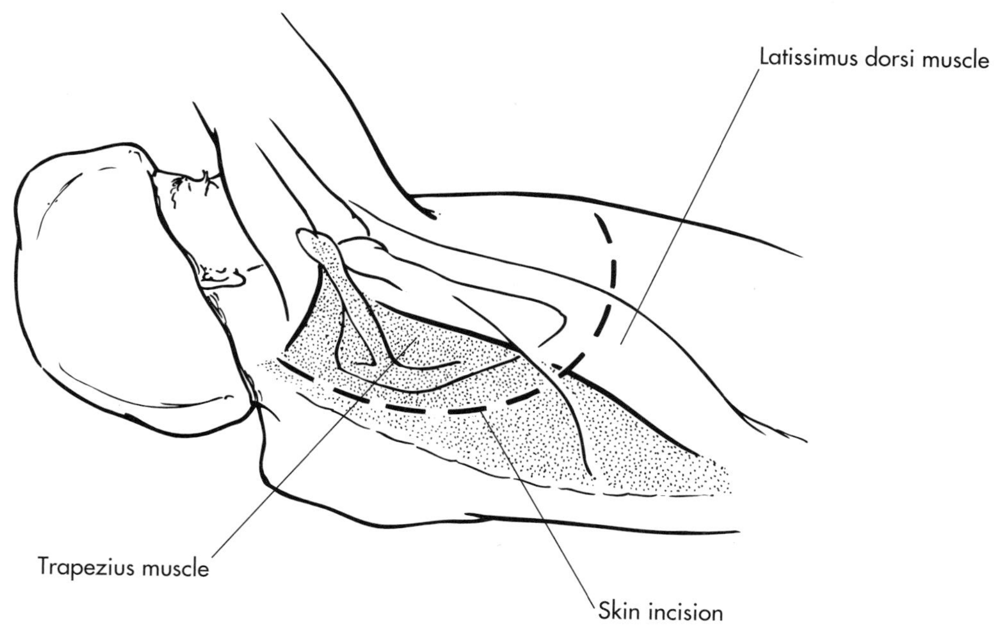

FIGURE 29-3

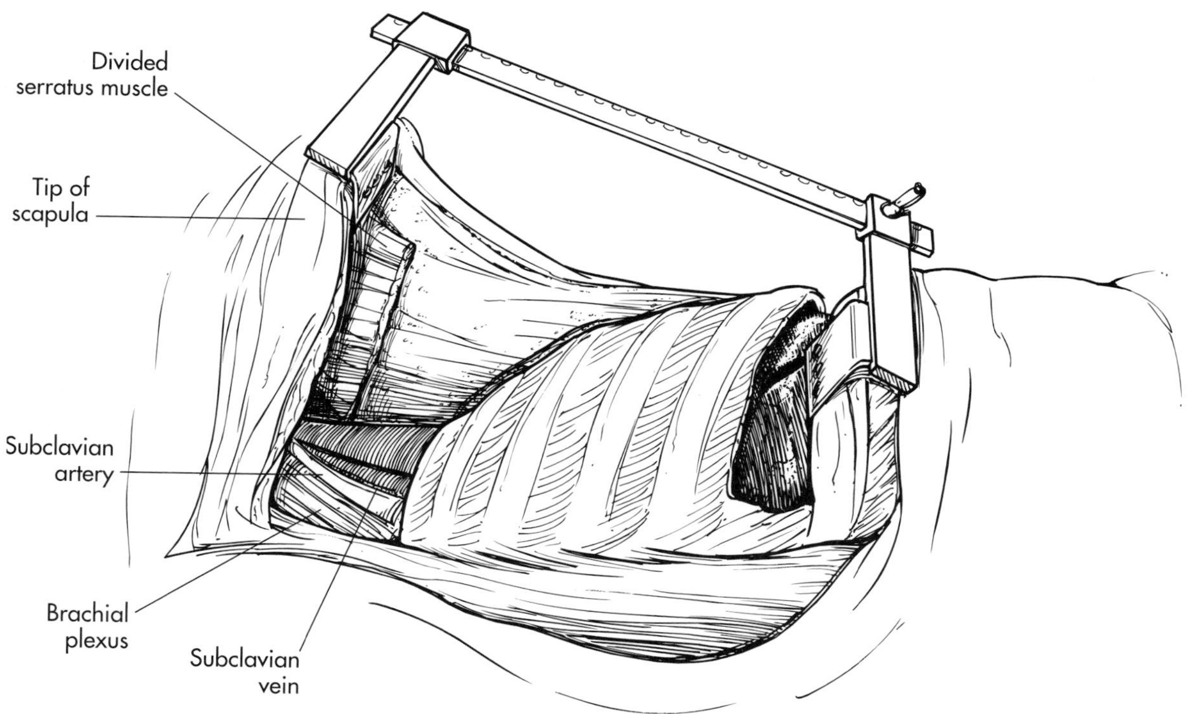

FIGURE 29-4

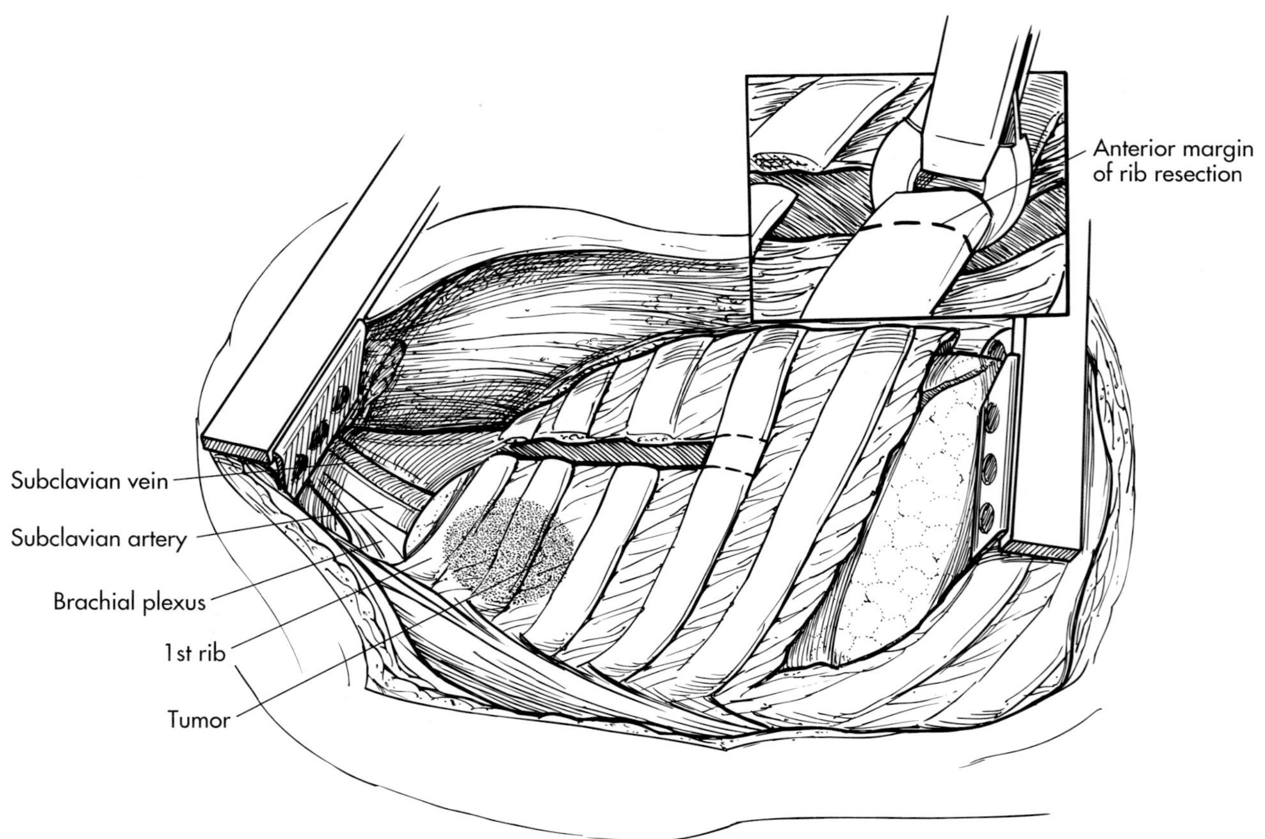

FIGURE 29-5

In most cases at least the first three ribs must be resected but depending on the extent of the tumor, more ribs might have to be taken. The inferior extent of the resection is assessed from within the chest, which has been entered through the 5th intercostal space. The resection is begun anteriorly on the inferior aspect of the block of chest wall to be resected. I begin the resection anteriorly by taking a 1- to 2-cm piece of rib at each level (**Fig. 29-5**). To do this the periosteum is incised and completely reflected off the piece of rib (**Fig. 29-5, *inset***). The piece of rib is cut and excised, which makes identification and ligation of the intercostal bundle easier as well as allows space for easier retraction of the chest wall block. Each piece of anterior rib is submitted to the pathologist separately as the anterior resection margin at each level. Because of the angles involved, special instruments designed for work on the first rib should be used at this level. These include several angled periosteal elevators and rib shears. The periosteal elevators should be used to skeletonize the first rib, removing any remnants of anterior or middle scalene muscle, and then the rib is encircled, with the surgeon taking care to stay directly on the rib so as to prevent injury to the subclavian vein or the brachial plexus. The artery may be dissected out so that it can be easily visualized. Once around the anterior aspect of the first rib, the anterior first rib cutter is used to cut the rib. This rib is usually flat and broad, and a considerable amount of power must be applied to the rib cutter to cut through it. No attempt is made to take a segment of this rib. The anterior portion of the resection is completed before the posterior part of the resection is done.

Posteriorly, the ribs must be disarticulated from the transverse process at each level. Depending on the extent of the tumor, it may be necessary as well to excise the transverse process. This posterior aspect of the resection is accomplished by reflecting the erector spinae ligament to expose the ribs back to the level of the transverse process. The transverse process at each level is easily palpated. There is a cartilaginous attachment between the neck of the rib and the transverse process that must be

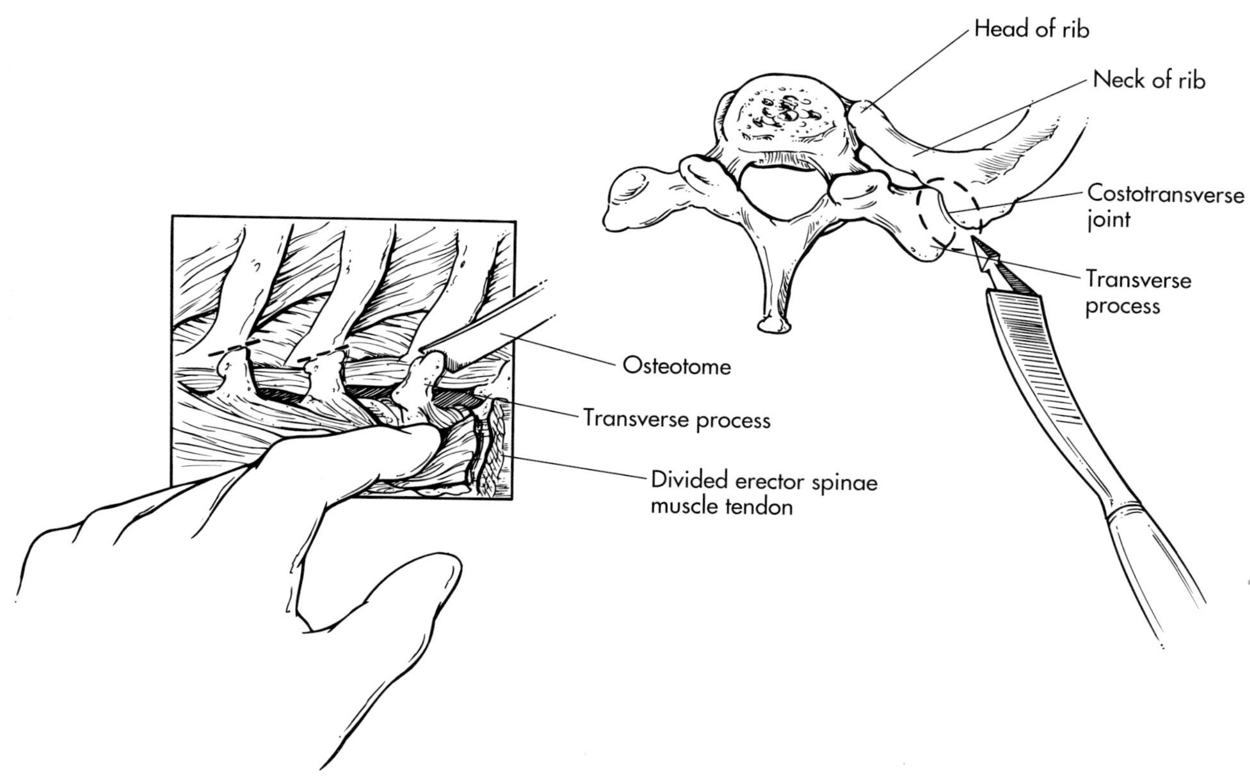

FIGURE 29-6

incised with electrocautery (**Fig. 29-6**). Once the correct location is found, this cartilaginous junction readily melts as the electrocautery is applied. An osteotome is then inserted between the rib and the transverse process, and force is applied in an anterior direction (**Fig. 29-6, *inset***). Gradually, the neck of the rib separates from the transverse process and the head of the rib from the vertebral body. This maneuver is facilitated if the parietal pleura overlying the head of the rib is incised. As each rib is disarticulated, the intercostal nerve and vessels must be identified, ligated, and divided. The nerve root must be ligated as it exits from the neural foramen. Avulsing a nerve root may result in a cerebrospinal fluid leak since the extent of the dural sheath on the nerve root is variable. Bleeding at the level of the neural foramen may be quite troublesome and should be controlled with careful use of bipolar cautery. Bone wax or Gelfoam should not be forced into the foramen, as they may result in spinal cord compression and paraplegia. A piece of Gelfoam applied to the foramen and covered with a dry sponge will go a long way to stopping most of this venous bleeding, but it is best to avoid creating bleeding in this area.

Taking the posterior aspect of the first rib is the most difficult and potentially dangerous part of the entire operation, though it is made somewhat easier by dividing the rib anteriorly, as we have already discussed. The first rib is skeletonized in a subperiosteal plane back to the transverse process. The first rib attaches to C7 and sits between the C8 and T1 nerve roots, and it is particularly important to carry the dissection back to this level (**Fig. 29-7**). If these roots are not seen as distinct structures exiting from their respective foramina, there is a chance of cutting the lower cord of the brachial plexus, with the surgeon thinking it is the T1 nerve root and leaving the patient with a useless hand. If involved with tumor, the T1 nerve root may be divided, usually with minimal sequelae, since its contribution to the ulnar nerve is relatively minor, though there is considerable individual variation in the extent of the contribution. Taking both the C8 and T1 nerve roots leaves the patient with a clawed hand, and if there is extensive involvement of the brachial plexus with tumor it is probably better to leave the nerve roots intact and refer the patient for radiation therapy, recognizing the dis-

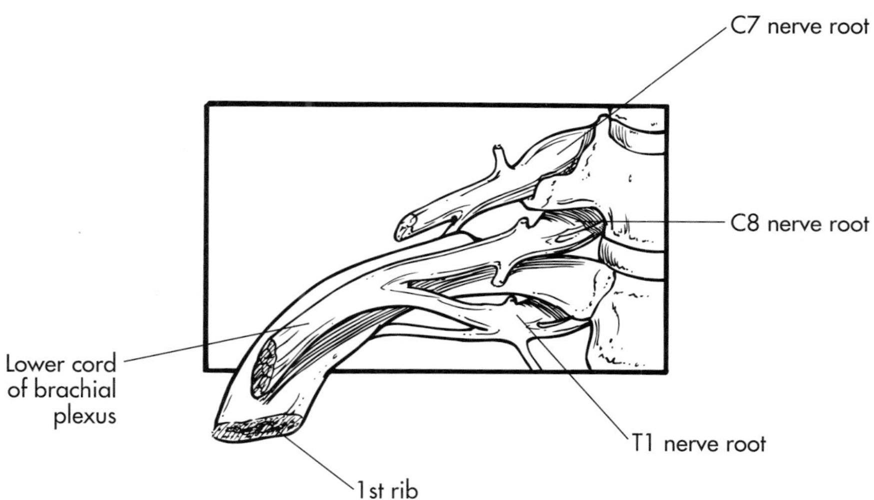

FIGURE 29-7

mal nature of such a lesion. The first rib is then cut with the posterior first rib cutter. If the subclavian artery is involved, a segment may be resected and reconstructed with vein graft or prosthetic material. Likewise, a segment of subclavian vein may be resected if required. Before resecting vessels, however, one should be certain that so doing will result in a complete resection, thus justifying the potential for greater morbidity.

Preoperatively, MRI scanning is useful in detecting vertebral body involvement, and extensive involvement at this level usually precludes resection. Even if resected, vertebral body involvement carries a very poor prognosis for long-term survival. If vertebral body involvement is identified at the time of resection, it is best to enlist a neurosurgeon who is willing to resect a portion or all of one or several vertebral bodies, if necessary. Not all neurosurgeons, however, are willing or able to participate in these procedures, a point that must be kept in mind when contemplating surgical intervention for these lesions.

Once the rib block has been entirely mobilized, a standard upper lobectomy is performed accompanied by a lymph node dissection, which completes the staging. With the first rib resected, the subclavian vessels and brachial plexus are nicely exposed (**Fig. 29-8**). If the resection has been confined to the first 3 ribs posteriorly, the entire defect will be covered by the scapula and there is no need for reconstruction of the chest wall with prosthetic material. If the 4th rib has been removed, there is a significant likelihood of the scapula "catching" on the edge of the 5th rib and getting caught within the chest, a situation particularly annoying to the patient. If the 4th rib has been resected, the chest wall defect is reconstructed with a piece of polypropylene mesh, as discussed in the section on chest wall tumors. Methylmethacrylate is not used for defects in this location since the scapula covers the majority of the defect.

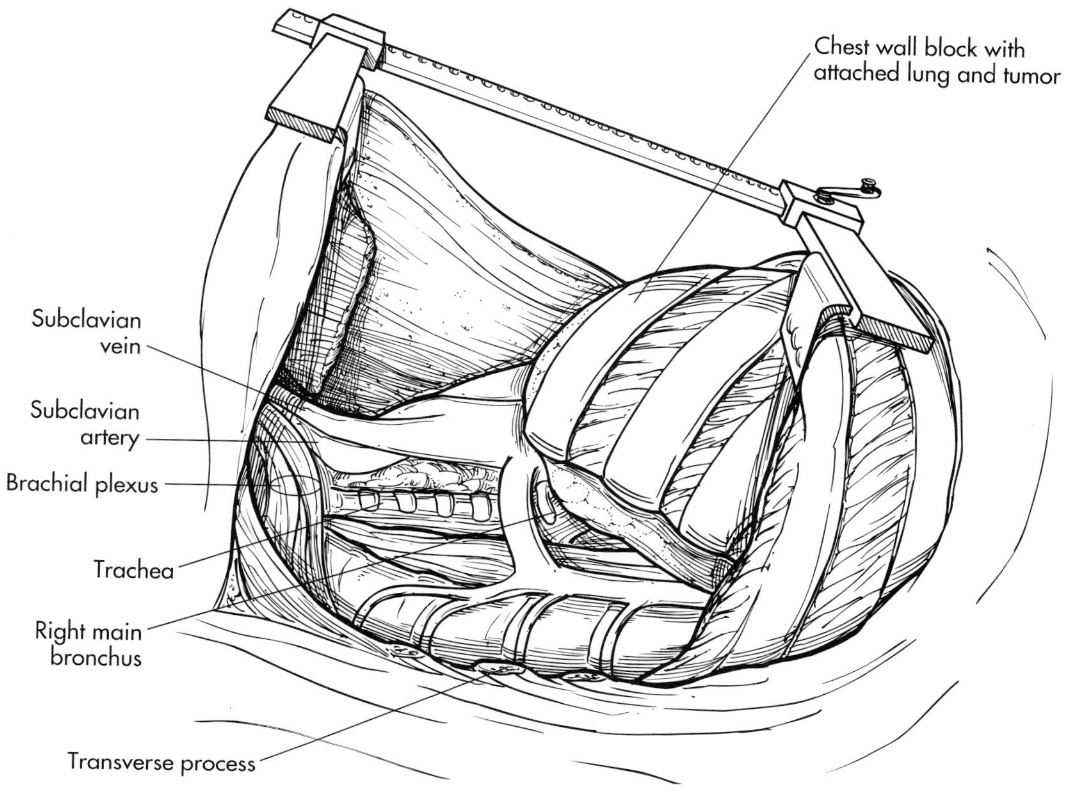

FIGURE 29-8

To close this extensive wound the trapezius muscle is reapproximated, a closure I perform with interrupted sutures if the patient has received preoperative radiation therapy; the serratus and latissimus muscles are approximated as is the subcutaneous tissue, and the skin is closed with skin staples. In the early postoperative period I place the ipsilateral arm in a sling for patient comfort. The need for additional postoperative therapy is dependent on findings at the operation.

Bibliography

Ginsberg RJ: Resection of a superior sulcus tumor, *Chest Surg Clin North Am* 5:315–331, 1995.

Komaki R, Mountain CF, Holbert JM, et al: Superior sulcus tumors: treatment selection and results for 85 patients without metastasis (M0) at presentation, *Int J Radiat Oncol Biol Phys* 19:31–36, 1990.

Neal CR, Amdur RJ, Mendenhall WM, et al: Pancoast tumor: radiation therapy alone versus preoperative radiation therapy and surgery, *Int J Radiat Oncol Biol Phys* 21:651–660, 1991.

Pancoast HK: Superior pulmonary sulcus tumors: tumor characterized by pain, Horner's syndrome, destruction of bone, and atrophy of hand muscles, *JAMA* 99:1391–1396, 1932.

PART VI

Miscellaneous Procedures

CHAPTER 30

Pleurectomy and Decortication

The management of the infected pleural space presents one of the more challenging problems faced by the thoracic surgeon. With the recent developments in thoracoscopy there has been a trend toward earlier drainage and débridement of the infected space with the hope of avoiding a larger procedure later. The fibrinous, almost gelatinous exudate found at thoracoscopic drainage early in the course of the infection organizes to become a fibrous peel encasing the lung later, often mandating pleurectomy and decortication.

The entire spectrum of residua following pleural space infections falls into the category of space problems, *space* here referring to areas within the hemithorax not filled by the expanded lung. Residual spaces, especially those that have been infected, are inherently evil to the chest surgeon. When the lung, entrapped by a fibrous peel, is unable to completely expand to fill the pleural space either in the presence of residual infection or as a consequence of a resolved infection, decortication may be indicated. We make a distinction between a subacute process where infected pleural contents, though organized as a fibrinous peel, are present and a chronic process where a firm, fibrous peel encases the lung. The intention of decortication is to remove the peel from the visceral pleural surface, allowing the lung to reexpand and fill the pleural space, thus obliterating any potential for an infected residual space.

Decortication usually is not indicated when the residual space is relatively small and well defined. In this situation, either rib resection and tube drainage or open window thoracostomy is the preferred procedure and each is discussed in a separate chapter. The judgment to proceed with decortication usually is based on a process that involves the pleural space diffusely. Timing is somewhat important, since an early organized pleural space infection may be managed with a videothoracoscopic approach (discussed in Chapter 8). In these early cases the peel usually is not completely organized, though it has solidified enough to make chest tube drainage ineffective. We handle these early cases preferentially with a video-assisted approach and open only when we deem it necessary based on what we observe with the videothoracoscope.

For open decortication of a subacute process where the peel is expected to be fairly solid and well organized, the chest is entered through a standard posterolateral thoracotomy incision (**Fig. 30-1**). I prefer to remove a rib since this facilitates an extrapleural dissection (pleurectomy), should this be required. Pleurectomy routinely is performed for chronic cases (>6 weeks in duration), since this allows better access to the chest and aids in cleaning out residual peel. Once the pleurectomy is performed, entry is made through the parietal pleura, which in many of these chronic cases is fused with the visceral pleura, and down onto the visceral pleural surface. If the parietal pleura is not fused with the visceral pleura, as is often the case in a subacute process, the adhesions between the visceral peel and the parietal pleura are taken down using a combination of sharp and blunt dissection (**Fig. 30-2**).

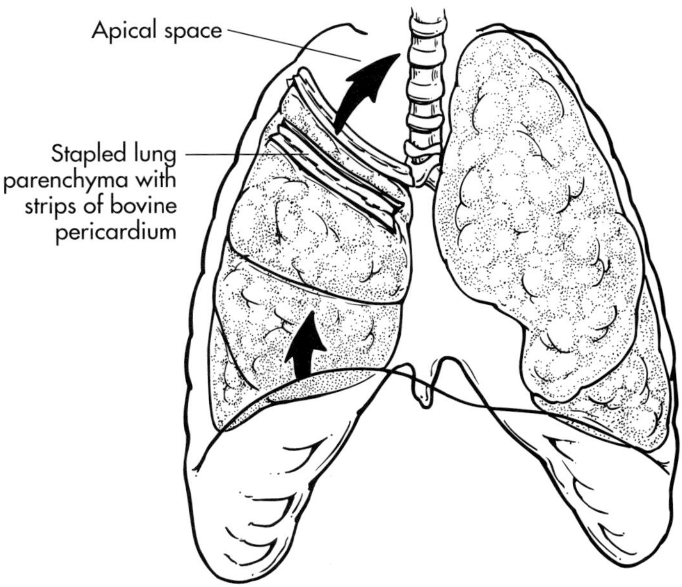

FIGURE 31-4

catheter is placed before induction of anesthesia and should be injected before the conclusion of the procedure. We avoid the use of long-acting narcotics in the epidural in this patient population and use instead local anesthetic. Good pulmonary toilet and secretion management are also extremely important.

This operation currently is undergoing critical evaluation in a number of centers. Long-term data are not yet available. Major questions that still remain to be answered include the duration of any benefit obtained and the definition of optimal criteria for patient selection. The procedure may also be accomplished via a videothoracoscopic approach with either both sides done under the same anesthetic or sequentially under different anesthetics. Results from a unilateral procedure have not been as consistently good as those seen when both sides are done. Whether it is possible to remove as much lung tissue through a videothoracoscopic approach compared to sternotomy remains to be determined. Also, whether there is any advantage to the thoracoscopic approach compared to sternotomy remains to be determined.

Bibliography

Cooper JD, Trulock EP, Triantafillou AN, et al: Bilateral pneumectomy (volume reduction) for chronic obstructive pulmonary disease, *J Thorac Cardiovasc Surg* 109:106-119, 1995.

Gaissert HA, Trulock EP, Cooper JD, et al: Comparison of early functional results after volume reduction or lung transplantation for chronic obstructive pulmonary disease, *J Thorac Cardiovasc Surg* 111:296-307, 1996.

CHAPTER 32

Transcervical Thymectomy

Excision of the thymus gland often plays a major role in the management of patients with myasthenia gravis. The exact relationship between this disease and the thymus gland and the reason why some patients go into remission after thymectomy remain unknown. Approximately 20% of patients with myasthenia gravis present with a tumor of the gland, a thymoma, which mandates excision as well as complete removal of the gland. The remainder of patients with the disease may benefit maximally from total thymectomy if it is done early in the course of the disease, though pharmacologic therapy with Mestinon remains the standard treatment. Older patients with the disease respond less well to thymectomy than younger patients. Often, the decision to perform thymectomy comes down to the beliefs and judgment of the individual neurologist. These patients are best managed by a neurologist who specializes in the care of patients with neuromuscular disease and ideally who has a particular interest in myasthenia gravis.

Classically, a median sternotomy is considered the standard approach for excision of the thymus gland, which in my judgment and that of a number of others is somewhat of a big operation for removal of what amounts to some well-encapsulated, almost avascular fatty tissue. Median sternotomy remains the procedure of choice when a thymoma is present, but transcervical thymectomy represents a viable alternative for patients with nonthymomatous glands. Neurologists always have been somewhat reluctant to refer patients for median sternotomy because of the magnitude of the operation, the possible complications relating to general anesthesia and neuromuscular blockade, and the possible difficulty of weaning these patients from the ventilator. Much of this reluctance tends to disappear with the realization that thymectomy may be performed through a neck incision, a significantly less invasive approach. This approach creates some objection and controversy within the surgical community because of the erroneous belief that total thymectomy cannot be accomplished because of problems presented by the variable location of portions of the gland. For the surgeon experienced in transcervical thymectomy, complete excision of the gland is the norm and the response rates for remissions have been comparable, though a prospective randomized study has never been done.

DESCRIPTION OF THE PROCEDURE

The patient is placed supine on the operating table with the neck maximally extended (**Fig. 32-1**). I use an inflatable bag placed behind the patient's shoulders to maximize the extension of the neck, since positioning is of extreme importance in the successful completion of this operation. The procedure is significantly more difficult in the patient whose neck cannot be hyperextended.

After a cosmetically acceptable transverse skin incision is outlined with a silk ligature 1 cm above the sternal notch, a cut is made and subplatysmal flaps are raised inferiorly down to the notch and superiorly to the thyroid cartilage. At the sternal notch the cleido-cleido ligament is incised with the

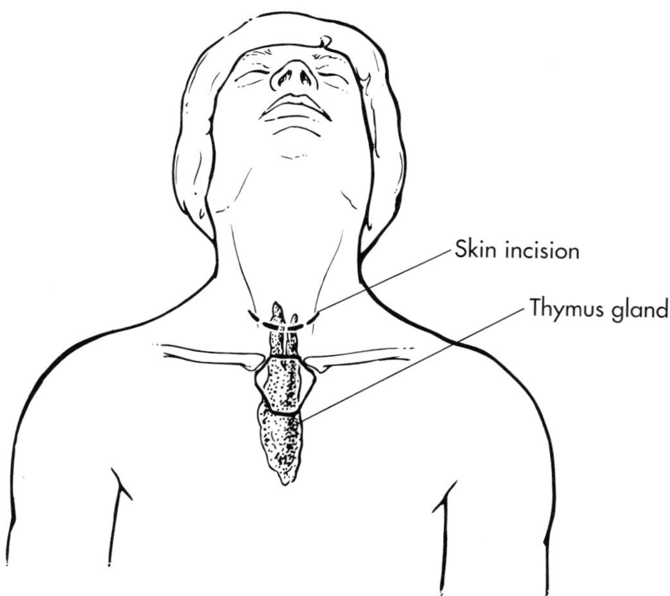

FIGURE 32-1

electrocautery and the small vein that usually is found in this area is coagulated. I insert a finger in the substernal plane to free the anterior mediastinal contents away from the posterior aspect of the sternum. Self-retaining retractors are placed, and dissection is begun along the midline. The sternohyoid muscles are separated in the midline but not divided. Dissection along the midline provides a relatively avascular plane.

The thymus gland is identified by developing a plane posterior to the sternothyroid muscle. It is sometimes difficult to distinguish the gland from the fat that is normally present, but the gland has a salmon pink color and a well-defined capsule. Identification of the gland may be especially difficult in the older patient where the gland is usually quite fatty. The inferior thyroid vein is used as a landmark, since the gland is located anterior to the vein. Usually the left lobe of the gland is identified first, since it frequently originates more superiorly in the neck than the right lobe. Once a lobe of the gland is identified, it is dissected up proximally to its origin. The gland thins out as one dissects farther proximally, but it is important to follow the gland as far proximally as possible. A silk tie is placed on the apex of the gland to use as a "handle" to manipulate the gland during the dissection (**Fig. 32-2**). The lobe of the gland that has been elevated is further mobilized by dissecting out the anterior, lateral, and medial aspects. With the surgeon following this lobe inferiorly and medially, the right lobe of the gland is identified, which is then similarly mobilized. A silk tie is placed around the apex of this lobe, and dissection proceeds farther inferiorly. Usually at this point, most of the mobilization occurs posterior to the gland down to the level of the innominate vein, which is easily visualized. Blunt dissection with a peanut sponge mounted on a hemostat is used to separate the gland from the innominate vein so as to identify venous branches draining the gland. Usually two or three venous branches are identified, and these are ligated with fine silk ligatures rather than the placing of metal clips, which are subject to dislodge with the further dissection required to complete the operation (**Fig. 32-3**). The lobes of the gland are retracted anteriorly, and a right-angle clamp is placed around the venous branch as the innominate vein is pulled posteriorly with the peanut sponge. The branch is ligated in continuity and divided. This is repeated for the other venous branches. The gland almost always resides anterior to the innominate vein, but occasionally a lobe or accessory lobe passes posterior to the vein. Discrete arterial branches to the gland requiring individual ligation are rarely identified, though occasionally one or two are seen laterally.

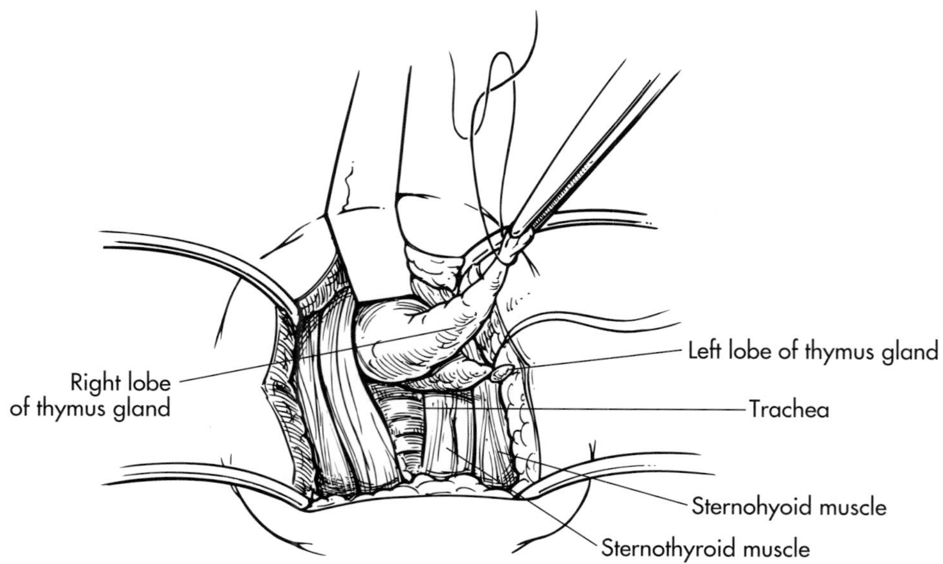
Left lobe of thymus gland
Right lobe
of thymus gland
Trachea
Sternohyoid muscle
Sternothyroid muscle

FIGURE 32-2

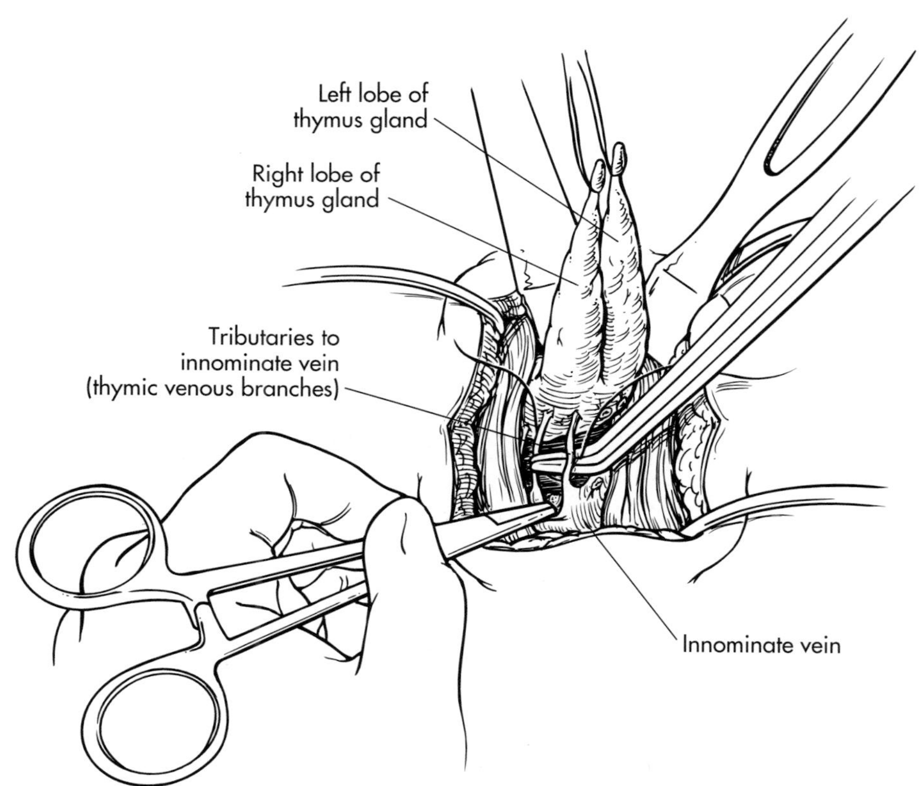
Left lobe of
thymus gland
Right lobe of
thymus gland
Tributaries to
innominate vein
(thymic venous branches)
Innominate vein

FIGURE 32-3

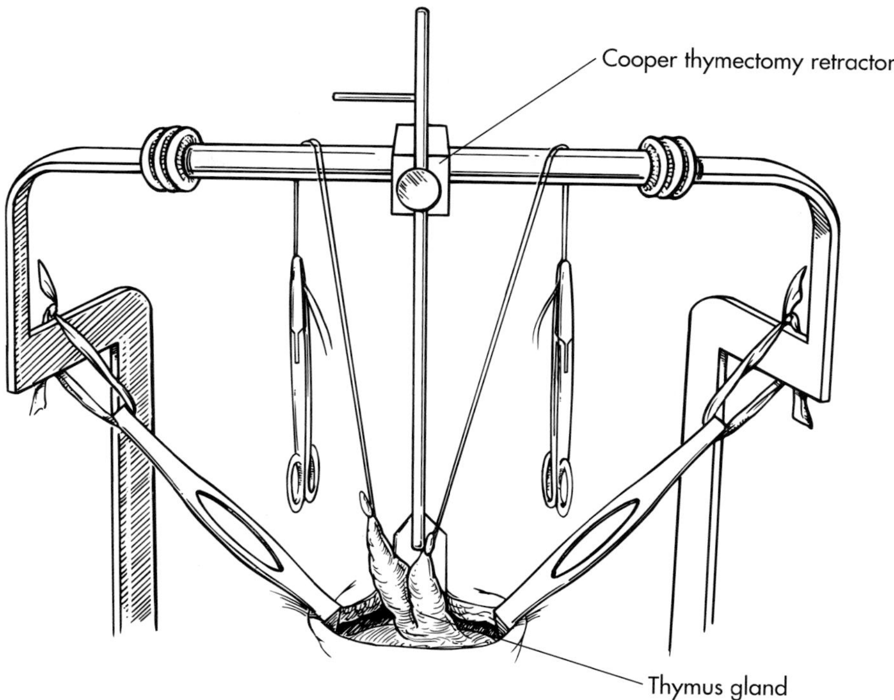

FIGURE 32-4

Once the venous branches have been divided, the gland is bluntly dissected completely off the innominate vein. Further mobilization is accomplished laterally using sharp dissection. The gland is retracted toward the right and the left lateral bands are incised and vice versa for the left lobe. At this point the thymectomy retractor (Cooper Thymectomy Retractor, Pilling-Weck, Research Triangle Park, N.C.) is put into place so that the rest of the anterior mediastinum is exposed. The side bars of the retractor are placed into the holders attached to the sides of the table and the crossbar is fitted on the retractor (**Fig. 32-4**). The blade is fitted onto the holder on the crossbar, then placed posterior to the sternal notch, this space having been defined by finger dissection. The blade is then forcefully lifted and secured in position, which essentially lifts the patient's head off the table. If the angle of placement of the retractor blade is even slightly off, the retractor will slip out of the sternal notch and have to be replaced. This is common, and often it takes two or three attempts to position the retractor in the right location. Sometimes an assistant is required to hold the blade in place to secure it. The inflatable bag is deflated, yielding maximal exposure to the anterior mediastinum. An Army-Navy type retractor is placed on each side of the wound, held in place by a Penrose drain tied to it and the side arms of the retractor (**Fig. 32-4**). Just enough tension should be applied by the Penrose drains to retract but not distort the edges of the wound.

Once the thymectomy retractor is in place, the surgeon sits on a stool at the head of the table at a comfortable height that allows for visualization down into the depths of the wound. This operation must be performed using a headlight and magnifying loupes are helpful. A headlight is absolutely mandatory, since there is no overhead light that provides enough illumination for so small of a hole that is of this depth. The remainder of the operation involves mobilizing the gland off the pleural reflections bilaterally, from the posterior aspect of the sternum, and from the pericardium. All of these areas are nicely visualized with the retractor in place as the dissection proceeds inferiorly. I accomplish much of this dissection bluntly using ball sponges (Tonsil Sponge Medium, Codman-Shurtleff Co.) placed on ring sponge forceps. One sponge is used for retraction and another sponge is used for mobilization of the gland off the pleural reflection (**Fig. 32-5**). This is done on both the right and left sides. The location of the phrenic nerves must be kept in mind to minimize the risk of

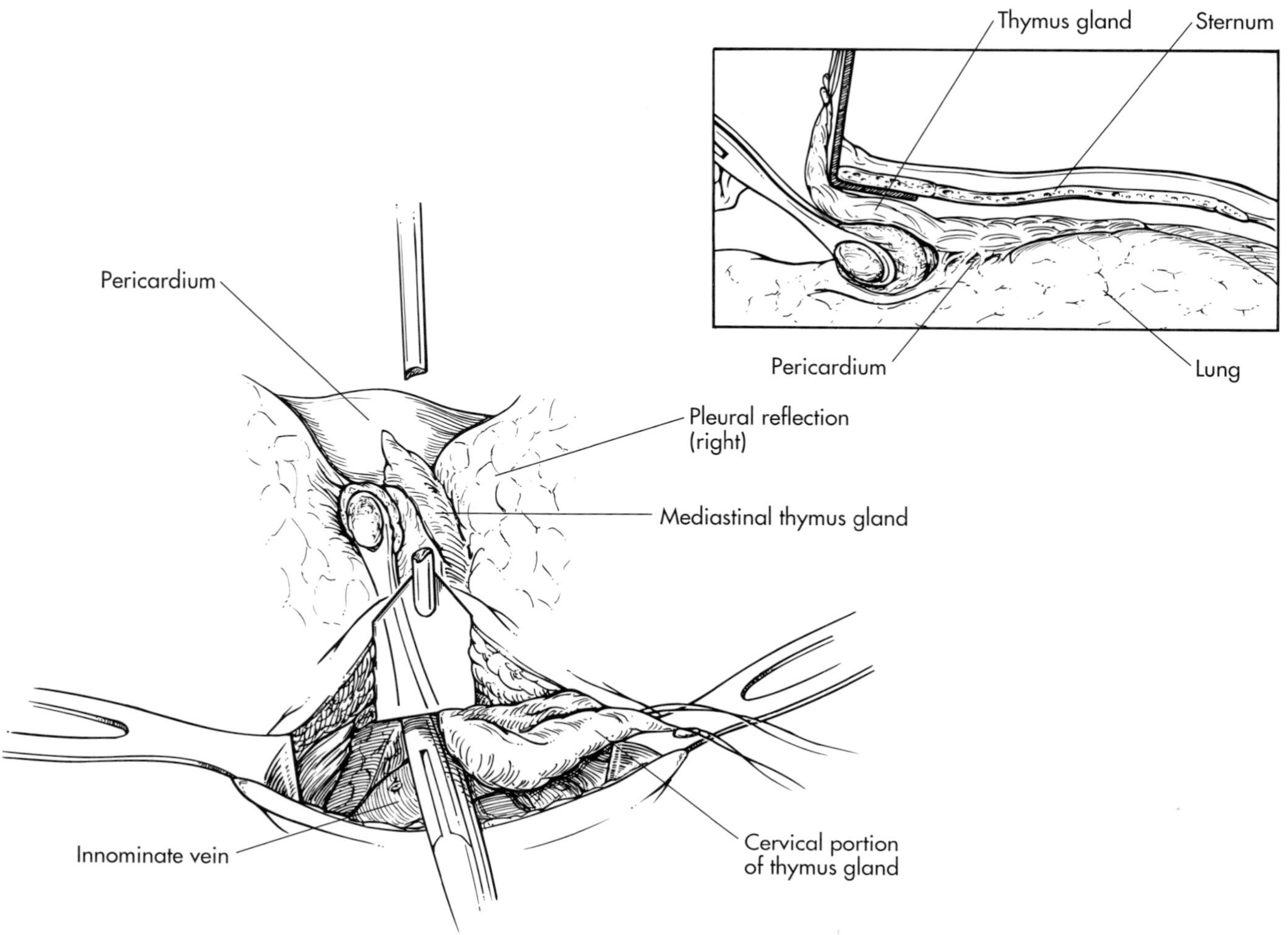

FIGURE 32-5

nerve injury, a complication that is significantly less likely to occur when using the blunt dissection technique described. There is usually a significant amount of fat on each pleural reflection, which is sometimes difficult to distinguish from the gland. I tend to take much of this fat if it dissects off with the gland, but it is often possible to visually distinguish between the gland and the pleural fat. If there is any doubt, all of the fatty tissue is taken. The occasional fibrous band must be divided sharply. The gland is also bluntly dissected off the pericardium, aided occasionally by incising a fibrous band (**Fig. 32-5, *inset***). Once the inferior extent of one lobe, usually the left, has been totally freed up, the rest of the mobilization of the gland is aided by pulling the gland upward toward the neck. We devote considerable attention to any aberrant location that might harbor glandular tissue, specifically the aortopulmonary window, which is readily accessible through this exposure. Eventually, the entire gland can be mobilized and delivered up into the neck.

The mediastinum is inspected for bleeding, and metal clips or the electrocautery is used to deal with any bleeding points. If a pleural space has been entered in dissecting the gland off a pleural reflection, a red rubber tube (Robinson) is placed into the open pleural space and brought up into the neck. The wound is closed in layers, first reapproximating the strap muscles, then the platysma. Once the platysma is closed, the anesthesiologist is asked to hold the lungs inflated and the rubber catheter is removed. A postoperative chest radiograph should be checked, but even if there is a small residual pneumothorax, I tend to do nothing since there is no ongo-

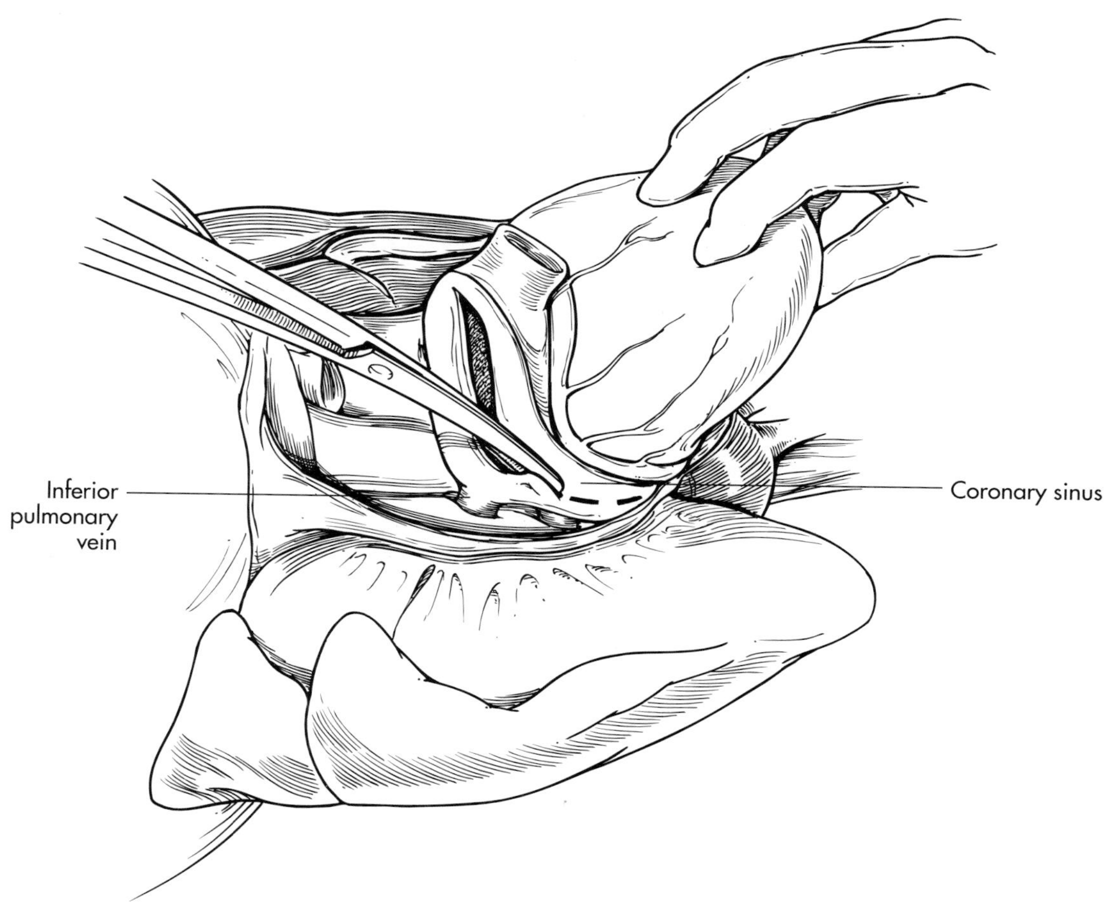

FIGURE 33-1

When 3 L of flush solution has been infused, the pulmonary artery is divided just proximal to the bifurcation. The venae cavae are divided as is the aorta. The heart is then retracted out of the chest, aimed in a direction pointing towards the right shoulder, and a cut is made in the left atrium midway between the coronary sinus and the entry of the left-sided pulmonary veins (**Fig. 33-1**). This allows for enough atrial cuff to be left with the heart so as not to compromise the cardiac graft and for enough cuff around the pulmonary venous remnants so that both lungs will be usable. The incision in the atrium proceeds superiorly, and the right-sided venous orifices are visualized from within the atrium. This allows for visualization of the cuff as it proceeds toward the right side. If the interatrial groove has been dissected, the cut proceeds along this line. The heart is removed after the atrial cut, and the dissection of the lung block proceeds. The innominate vein is divided, and the posterior pericardium is incised to reveal the trachea. The lungs are inflated to 30 cm H_2O pressure as the endotracheal tube is pulled back, and the trachea is stapled with a linear stapler. The esophagus is also stapled and divided at this level.

The pleural spaces are filled with iced saline solution to keep the lungs cool while the dissection proceeds. The right and left inferior pulmonary ligaments are divided, and the esophagus is stapled and divided at the level of the diaphragmatic hiatus. The right lung is retracted toward the left, and the pleura along the vertebral bodies is incised until the lung bloc is free. This allows the lungs to be removed en bloc with the esophagus, aorta, and posterior pericardium.

To prepare the lungs for implantation, the surgeon must excise the aorta and esophagus. This usually requires the aid of an assistant since the inflated lungs make this dissection somewhat difficult.

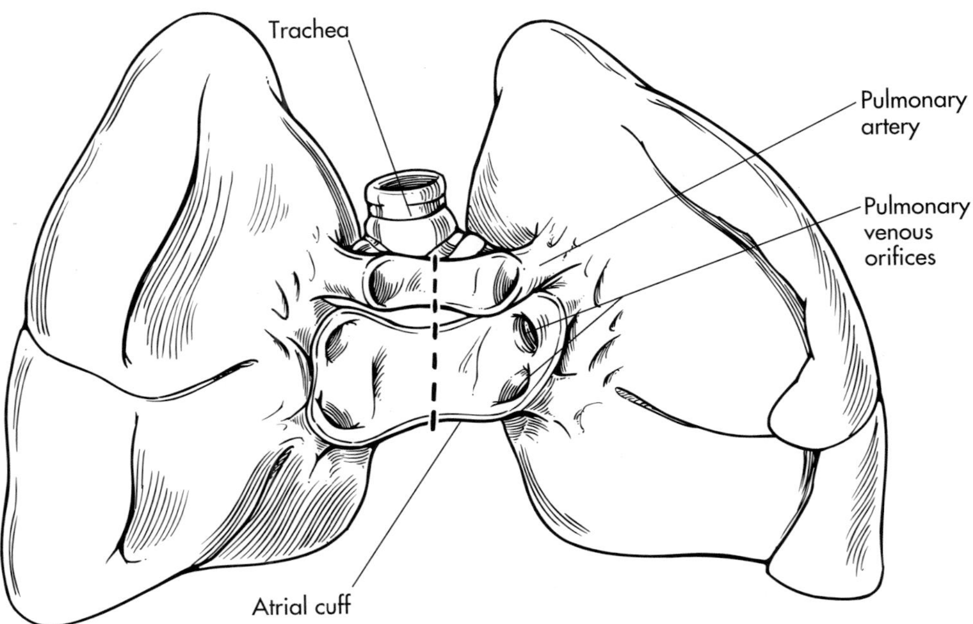

FIGURE 33-2

The aorta is separated from the pulmonary artery by dividing the ligamentum arteriosum. The pulmonary artery is divided at the bifurcation, and the artery to each lung is dissected free of the surrounding tissue (**Fig. 33-2**). The atrial cuff is divided into two, and the pericardium that remains with the block is excised. The right main stem bronchus is divided initially at the carina, and subsequently additional rings are taken so as to leave only two rings proximal to the right upper lobe takeoff. The left main bronchus is also trimmed to leave only two rings proximal to the bifurcation. The lungs are left immersed in iced saline solution, with care taken to avoid filling the bronchus with solution. The lungs are now ready for either single implantation or part of a bilateral sequential procedure.

Bibliography

Sundaresan S, Trachiotis G, Aoe M, et al: Donor lung procurement: assessment and operative technique, *Ann Thorac Surg* 56:1409–1413, 1993.

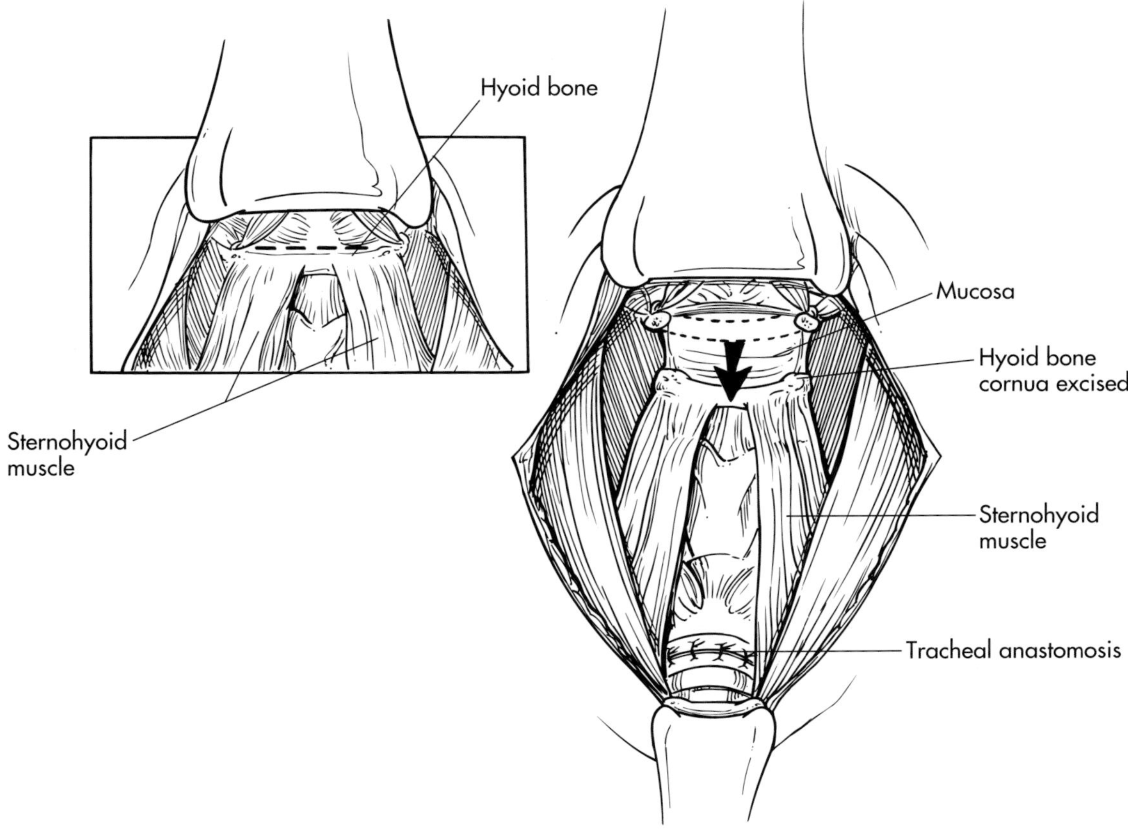

FIGURE 35-7

to remind the patient to avoid neck extension. This chin stitch is kept in place for 1 week. The endotracheal tube should be removed as soon as the patient is fully awake. If for any reason the tube needs to be replaced, it should be done with bronchoscopic guidance and not by lifting the larynx with a laryngoscope. After laryngeal release, swallowing may prove difficult initially for some patients and aspiration precautions must be taken. This problem occurs less after supralaryngeal release but is occasionally seen.

Bibliography

Bisson A, Bonnette P, el Kadi NB, et al: Tracheal sleeve resection for iatrogenic stenosis (subglottic laryngeal and tracheal), *J Thorac Cardiovasc Surg* 104:882–887, 1992.

Grillo HC and Mathisen DJ: Primary tracheal tumors: treatment and results, *Ann Thorac Surg* 49:69–77, 1990.

Mansour KA, Lee RB, Miller JI Jr: Tracheal resections: lessons learned, *Ann Thorac Surg* 57:1120–1124, 1994.

PART IX

The Esophagus

CHAPTER 36

Excision of Zenker's Diverticulum: Cricopharyngeal Myotomy

A cricopharyngeal diverticulum, by definition, is not a true diverticulum since not all layers of the esophagus are involved. This "diverticulum" results from disordered motility, namely high cricopharyngeal pressures not in coordination with initiation of swallowing. Instead of the cricopharyngeus relaxing upon initiation of swallowing, there is a delay in relaxation, causing high pressures to be exerted on the wall of the pharynx and esophagus. In the long term an outpouching of the mucosa at the weakest point, the junction between the inferior pharyngeal constrictor and the cricopharyngeus, occurs. Initially it is asymptomatic. As this outpouching increases in size, gurgling upon swallowing is noted and undigested food may be regurgitated. Aspiration pneumonia or evidence of chronic aspiration may be seen in some cases. The treatment for this problem must be directed at the underlying pathologic process, the motility disorder, not solely at the diverticulum. If the diverticulum only is excised, recurrence can be expected over time. In fact, the diverticulum does not even need to be excised but can be inverted with its opening diverted away from the flow down the esophagus so long as the motility disorder is addressed with a myotomy.

DESCRIPTION OF THE PROCEDURE

The patient is placed on the operating table in the supine position with the neck hyperextended. An inflatable bag placed behind the patient's shoulders maximally extends the neck. Preferentially, the procedure is performed via the left side of the neck because of the more constant course of the recurrent laryngeal nerve, which remains closer to the tracheoesophageal groove than it does on the right side. The chance of recurrent laryngeal nerve injury is lessened by operating on the left side of the neck. A skin incision is made along the anterior border of the sternocleidomastoid muscle and deepened through the subcutaneous tissue. Dissection proceeds along the anterior border of the sternocleidomastoid medial to the carotid sheath down to the prevertebral fascia. The omohyoid muscle should be divided to enhance the exposure. In most cases the diverticulum is not immediately obvious. In fact, even those that appear large on radiographic studies are often difficult to identify in the anesthetized patient. Usually, the diverticulum is adherent to the cricopharyngeus and is difficult to see when decompressed.

The larynx is retracted toward the right to expose the pharyngeal constrictors and the cricopharyngeus (**Fig. 36-1**). This retraction is best accomplished with the assistant's finger, though an angled retractor may be used as long as care is taken to avoid retraction of the tracheoesophageal groove where the recurrent laryngeal nerve resides. Once the junction between the inferior constrictor and the cricopharyngeus is seen, the diverticulum should be reasonably easy to identify and mobilize since it originates from this point of weakness (***see* Fig. 36-1**). The procedure may be facilitated by placing a 40-Fr bougie in the esophagus. The myotomy is begun at the junction between the inferior constrictor and the cricopharyngeus (**Fig. 36-2**). The plane is readily seen, since the

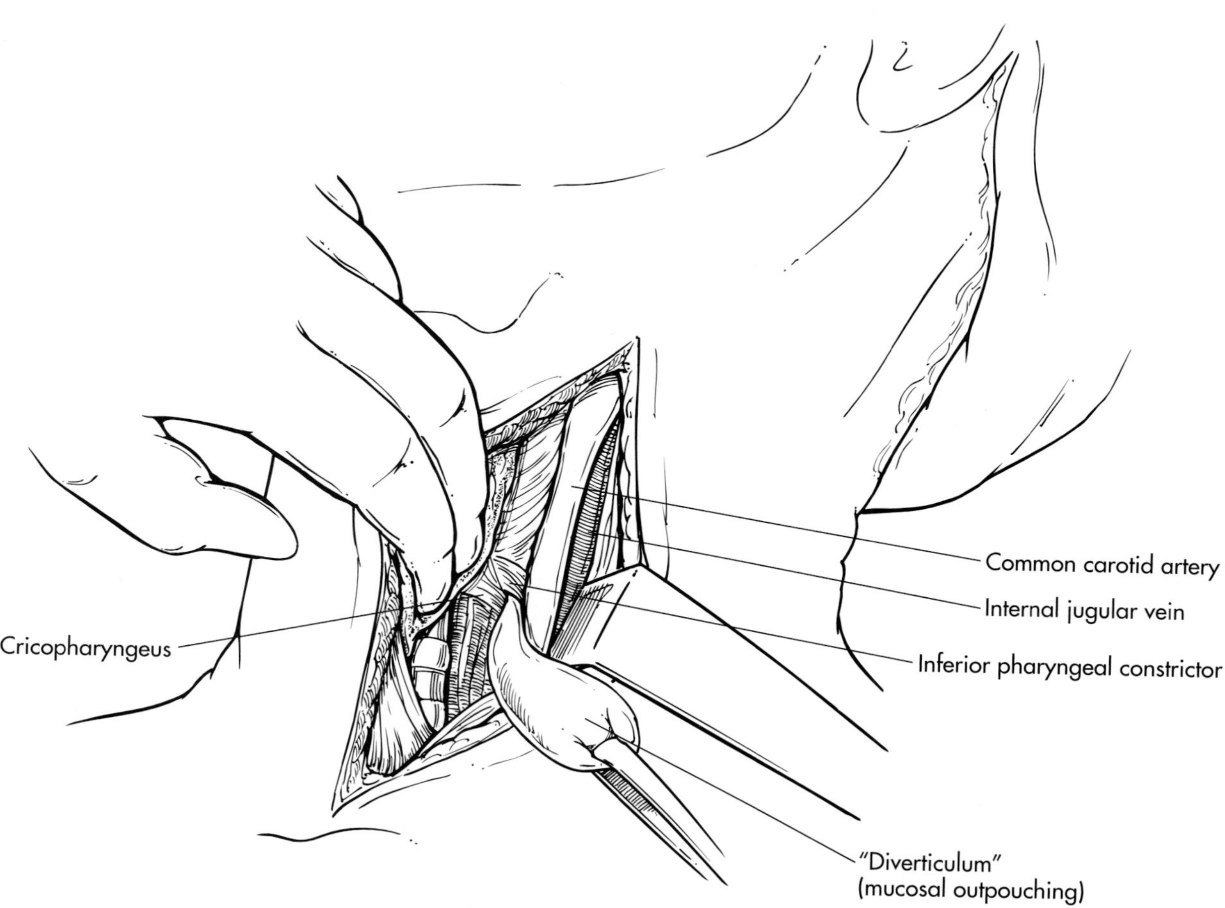
Common carotid artery
Internal jugular vein
Inferior pharyngeal constrictor
Cricopharyngeus
"Diverticulum"
(mucosal outpouching)

FIGURE 36-1

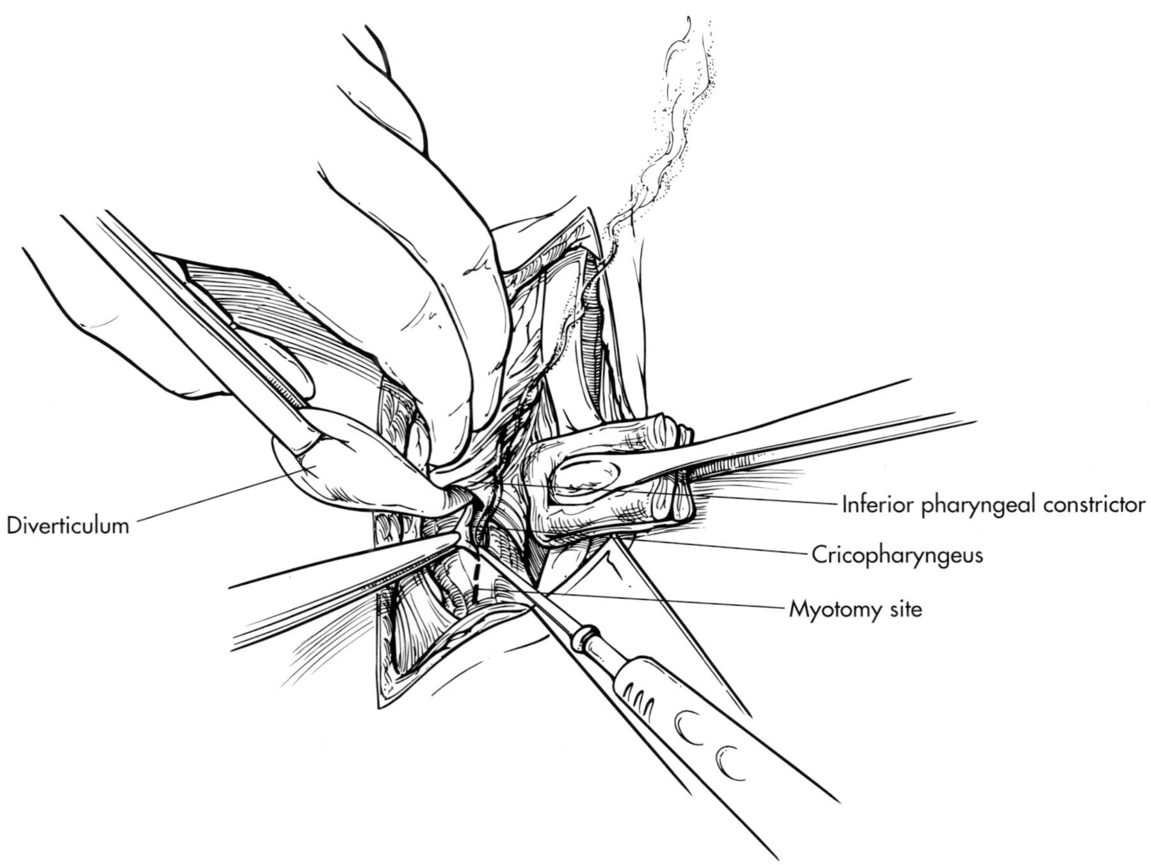

FIGURE 36-2

diverticulum is only mucosa and thus defines the plane. Either the cautery or, preferably, a scissors is used to incise both the longitudinal and circular layers of muscle extending down onto the esophagus (**Fig. 36-3**). A blunt right-angle clamp may be used to initially define the plane before incising.

In most cases I perform a diverticulopexy where the diverticulum is inverted and sewn to the prevertebral fascia, which functionally excludes the opening from the direction of food transit (**Fig. 36-3**). This eliminates the potential problem of stricture if too much mucosa is taken when excising the diverticulum and avoids a suture or staple line on the esophageal mucosa and the potential complications that accompany a leak from a hollow organ. Very large diverticula may require excision, but this would be an unusual situation. Some surgeons prefer to routinely excise a cricopharyngeal diverticulum. Excision should be carried out with a bougie in place to avoid taking too much mucosa and creating a stricture. A linear stapler may be fired across the base of the diverticulum, or it may be excised and sewn closed with interrupted sutures (**Fig. 36-3, *inset***). A closed suction drain should be left in place.

Patients who have had diverticulopexy may resume oral feedings on the day of operation, and those having excision should not resume eating for 2 to 3 days. Before removal of the suction drain,

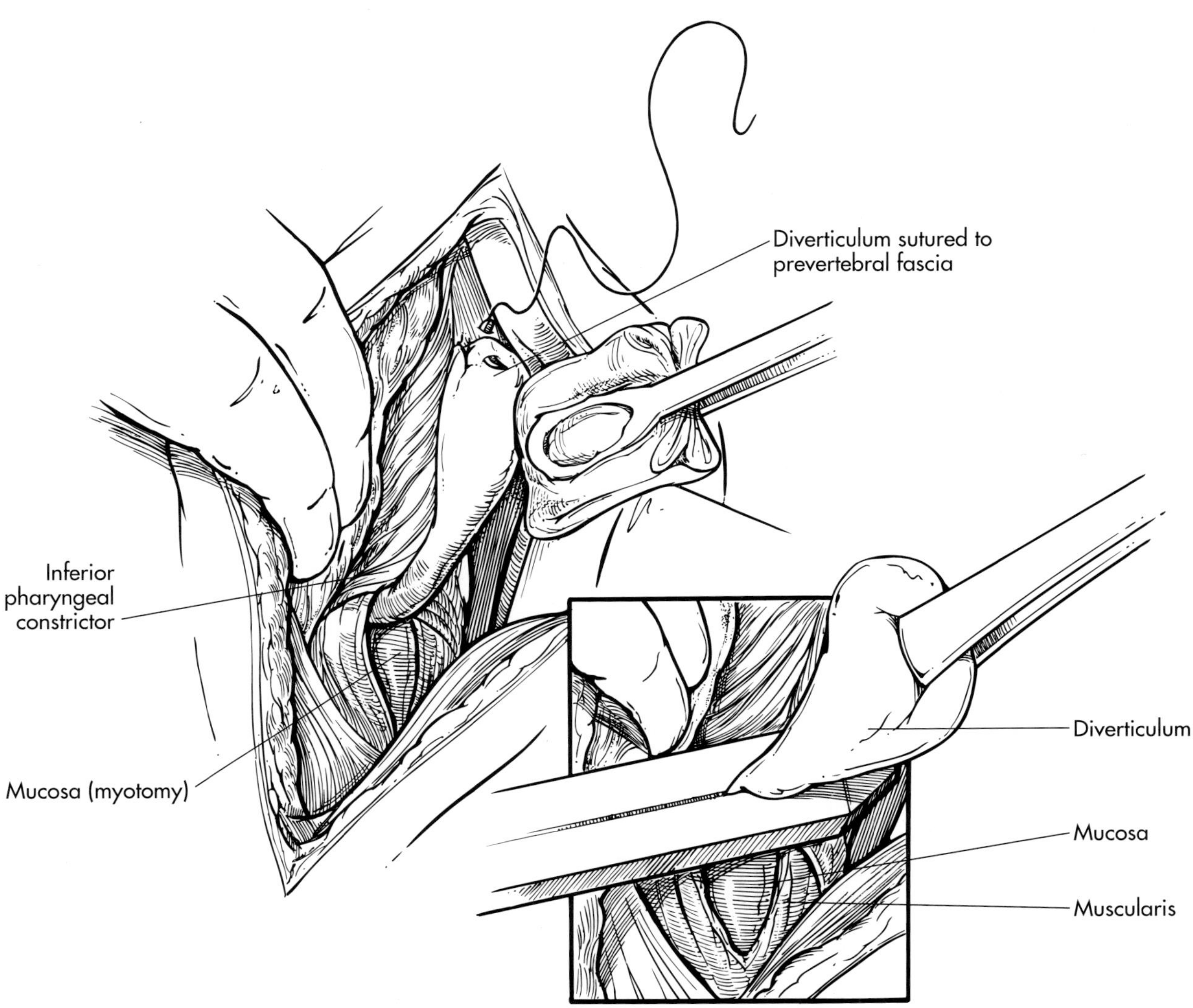

FIGURE 36-3

the patient may be given grape juice to see if any appears in the drainage collection unit. With no evidence of a leak the drain may be removed and the diet advanced.

Recurrence is rare after cricopharyngeal myotomy and is not dependent on whether diverticulopexy or excision was performed. Treatment of the motility problem is the key to success with this procedure.

Bibliography

Allen MS: Pharyngoesophageal diverticulum: technique of repair, *Chest Surg Clin North Am* 5:449–458, 1995.

Skinner DB, Altorki N, Ferguson M, et al: Zenker's diverticulum: clinical features and surgical management, *Diseases of the esophagus* 1:19–22, 1988.

CHAPTER 37

Esophageal Myotomy

Esophageal myotomy is performed mainly for achalasia, the most common primary motility disorder of the esophagus with an incidence of 6 per 100,000 individuals. The disease is characterized by an abnormal lower esophageal sphincter and almost complete absence of peristalsis in the esophageal body. The diagnosis is suspected based on radiographic findings seen on barium swallow and confirmed by motility testing. The classic finding on motility testing is abnormal relaxation of the lower esophageal sphincter and "mirror imaging" of the minimal peristaltic activity present. These patients usually are managed by pneumatic dilatation and come to operation only when dilatation fails or there is a complication from the dilatation procedure. Esophageal myotomy may also be done for the rare patient with diffuse esophageal spasm who fails medical management.

DESCRIPTION OF THE PROCEDURE

The operation is done through a left thoracotomy, though it has occasionally been performed via laparotomy. Recently, a video-assisted thoracoscopic technique has been described that avoids formal thoracotomy and results in the same outcome, at least with short-term follow-up, as the open technique. Whether visualization is accomplished via thoracotomy or a video-assisted approach, the myotomy is performed the same way and to the same extent. The chest is entered through the sixth intercostal space, and the esophagus is mobilized at the diaphragmatic hiatus (**Fig. 37-1**). The peri-

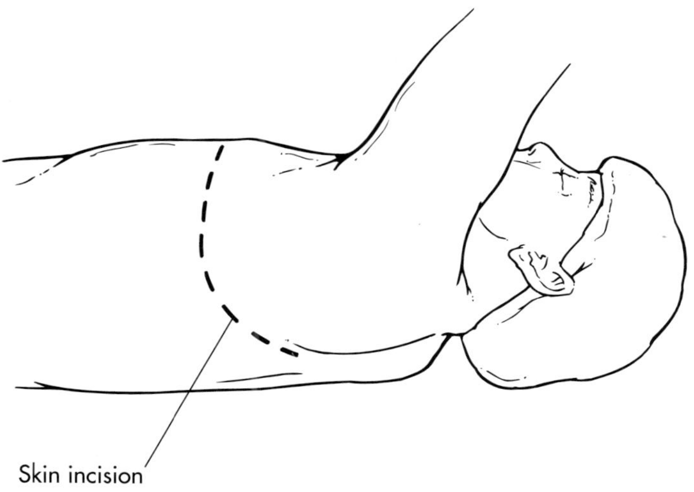

FIGURE 37-1

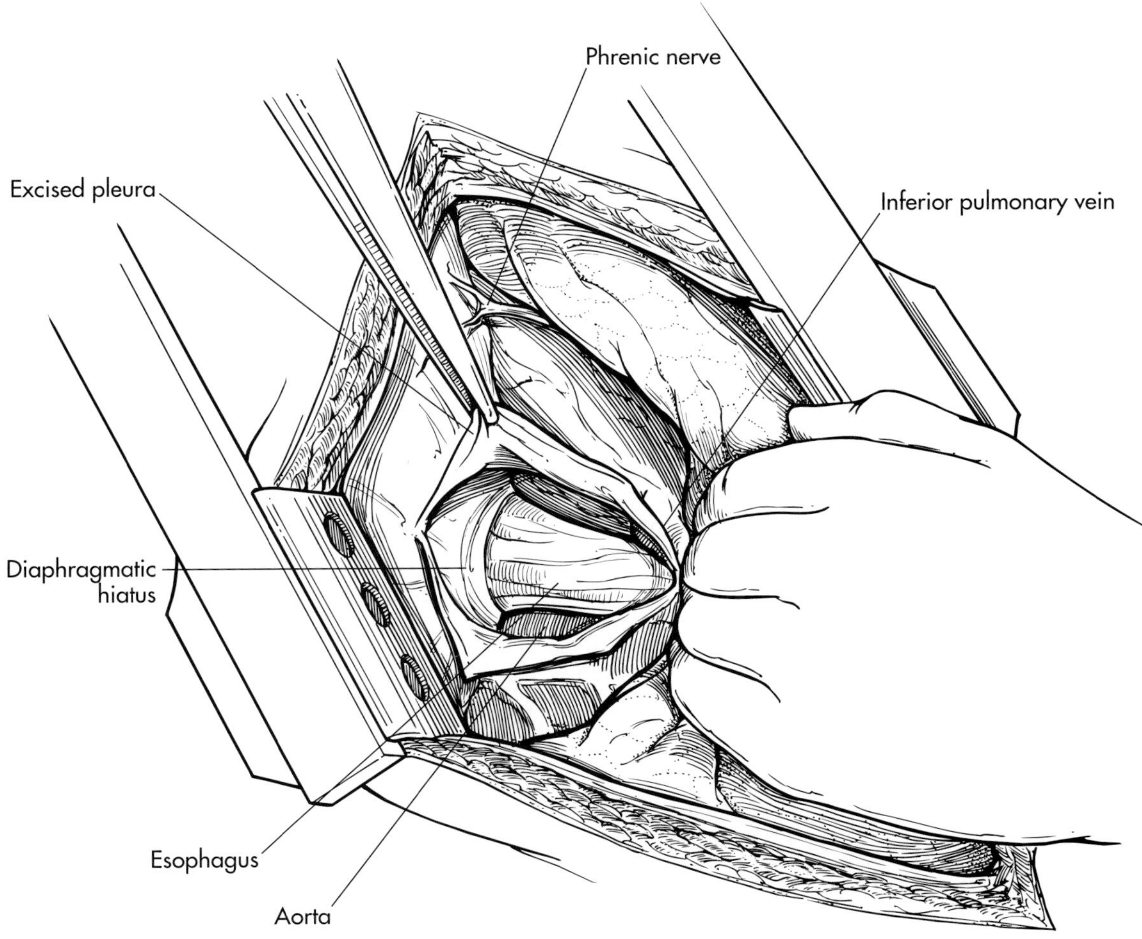

FIGURE 37-2

cardium is grasped with a Kocher clamp for traction, and dissection begins immediately adjacent to the pericardium until the esophagus is identified (**Fig. 37-2**). The esophagus routinely is mobilized up to the level of the inferior pulmonary vein or to the level of the aortic arch, if the procedure is being done for diffuse esophageal spasm. The hiatus is incised so that the stomach is visualized.

With the left hand placed behind the esophagus to lift it up and out of the mediastinum, thereby putting it under some tension, a blunt-tipped scissors is used to incise the longitudinal muscle (**Fig. 37-3**). Just deep to this layer the circular muscle is incised and the mucosa is then visualized (**Fig. 37-3, *inset***). Using a blunt-tipped scissors and cutting with the tips of the scissors directed perpendicular to the muscle safely allows the muscle to be cut, revealing each layer as the cut is made. The key is holding the esophagus under sufficient tension to facilitate the cut. A scalpel may also be used to make this initial cut but does not provide the degree of control afforded by the scissors. Once the plane of the mucosa is established, a right-angle clamp may be inserted deep to the circular muscle and used as a guide to extend the myotomy with the scissors. The myotomy should extend at least up to the level of the inferior pulmonary vein in patients with achalasia and up to the level of the aortic arch in diffuse esophageal spasm and down to just beyond the gastroesophageal junction (**Fig. 37-4**).

As the myotomy is extended distally, it becomes obvious when the cut has traversed the stomach, as bleeding from the submucosal gastric plexus of veins is distinctly different from any bleeding encountered when incising esophageal muscle. The cut should extend just onto the stomach as the gastric venous plexus becomes apparent. Extending the myotomy further onto the stomach results in

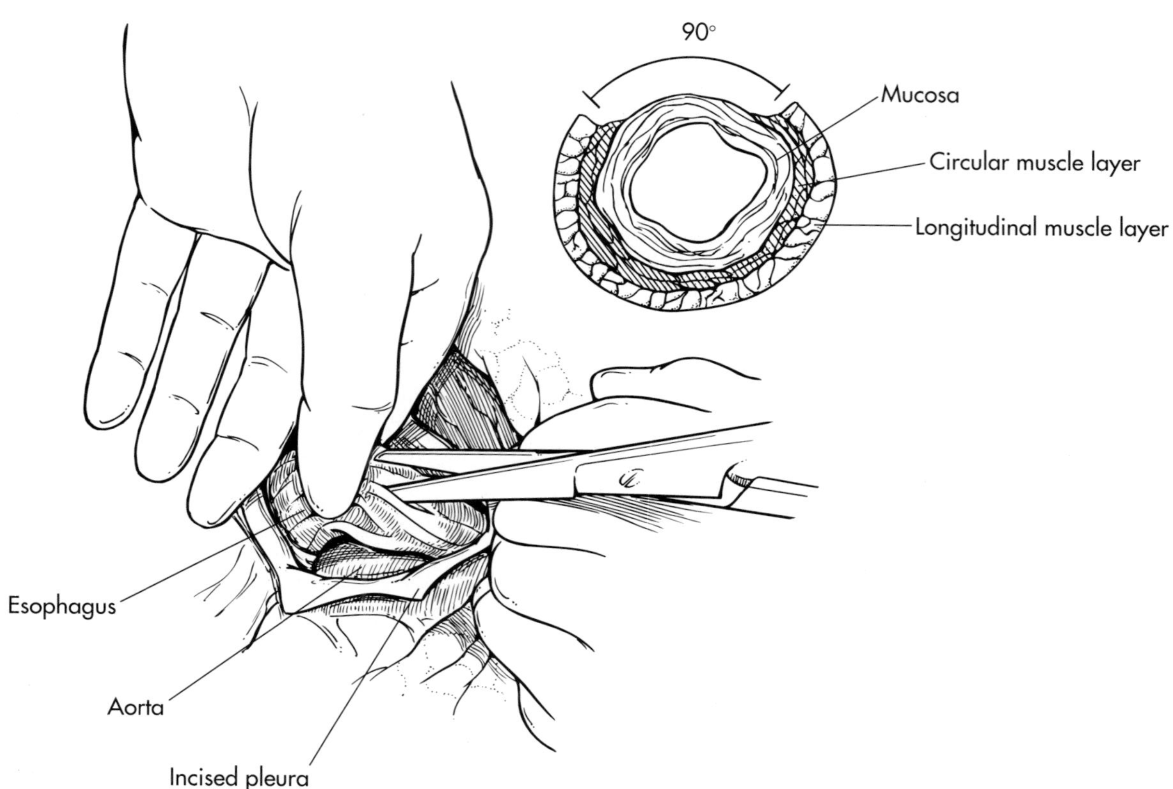
90°
Mucosa
Circular muscle layer
Longitudinal muscle layer
Esophagus
Aorta
Incised pleura

FIGURE 37-3

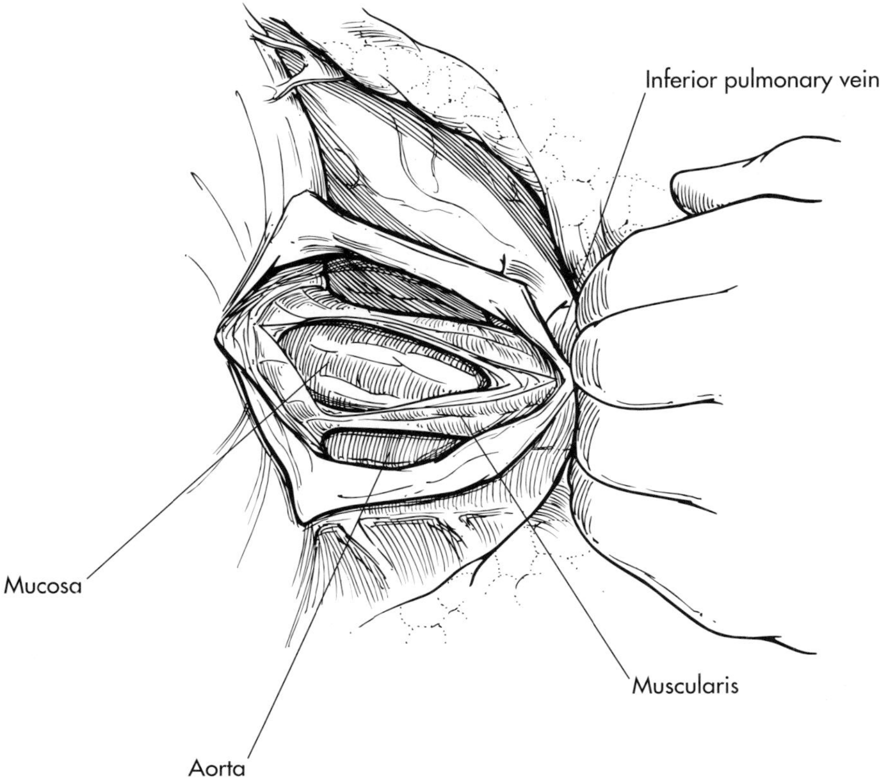

FIGURE 37-4

significant gastroesophageal reflux and the need for an antireflux procedure. There are a number of surgeons who feel that an antireflux procedure should be performed routinely with a myotomy, but this remains an area of considerable dispute. If during the preoperative evaluation the patient has been shown to have significant gastroesophageal reflux by the 24-hour pH study, then it is prudent to combine an antireflux procedure with the myotomy. Otherwise, the myotomy alone is performed without a concomitant antireflux procedure. Placing a wrap around an amotile esophagus invites trouble if the wrap is too snug or efficient. This introduces an entirely new set of problems that are best avoided if possible.

The edges of the divided esophageal muscle should be undermined so that there is at least 90 degrees of the circumference of the esophagus with exposed mucosa (***see* Fig. 37-3, *inset***). This should prevent the edges of the muscle from reapproximating. If the mucosa is inadvertently entered, the rent should be closed with interrupted fine silk sutures and the muscle closed over it with another layer of interrupted sutures. Another myotomy should be fashioned 180 degrees opposite to the first attempt.

A single chest tube is placed, and the wound is closed in the usual fashion. The tube may be removed on the first postoperative day following an uncomplicated myotomy; it should be left in place longer if the mucosa has been entered.

Esophageal myotomy is a procedure that lends itself well to a video-assisted approach. The myotomy that can be performed with thoracoscopic visualization is equivalent to that performed via the open procedure. The monitor is placed at the foot of the operating table, and the videothoracoscope is inserted in the 7th intercostal space aligned with the anterosuperior iliac spine. Additional incisions are placed just inferior to the scapular tip in the 5th intercostal space and posterior in the 7th or 8th space. With a flexible esophagoscope in place to provide internal visualization and traction, the pleura overlying the esophagus is incised. With a curved instrument placed in the inferior thoracoscopy port, the diaphragm is retracted downward so as to expose the hiatus, which is incised while the traction is maintained. The esophageal longitudinal muscle and circular muscle are incised as described previously, made easier because of the magnification afforded by the videothoracoscope. The long-term results of the thoracoscopic procedure need to be validated against those obtained by the open procedure before we can make the recommendation that myotomy should be performed routinely through a video-assisted approach.

After a myotomy the patient should note less food sticking, but swallowing is never perfect. Esophageal motility is still disordered, and the esophagus really acts more like a passive conduit than a peristaltic pump.

Bibliography

Arreola-Risa C, Sinanan M, and Pellegrini CA: Thoracoscopic Heller's myotomy: treatment of achalasia by the videoendoscopic approach, *Chest Surg Clin North Am* 5:459–469, 1995.

Ellis FHJ: Oesophagomyotomy for achalasia: a 22-year experience, *Br J Surg* 80:882–885, 1993.

Ferguson MK: Achalasia: correct evaluation and therapy, *Ann Thorac Surg* 52:336–342, 1991.

CHAPTER 38

Transhiatal Esophagectomy

Some have referred to the transhiatal esophagectomy as blunt esophagectomy, but essentially the entire procedure is done under direct vision. Only in the region of the carina is the visualization limited, and a portion of the dissection is done without benefit of direct vision. Because of this limitation, I prefer to use the transhiatal approach for lesions of either the proximal or distal esophagus but not for lesions of the midesophagus where dissection around the region of the carina represents the most significant aspect of the procedure. This underscores the importance of versatility on the part of the esophageal surgeon. No single operation is appropriate for all patients with esophageal cancer. There are several different approaches to esophagectomy, and it is necessary for the complete esophageal surgeon to be a master of all of them to best tailor the approach to the specific situation. That being said, clearly there are surgeons who favor transhiatal esophagectomy for almost all lesions because of the perceived advantage accrued by avoiding thoracotomy.

DESCRIPTION OF THE PROCEDURE

The patient is placed on the operating table in the supine position with the neck hyperextended and the head turned to the right to expose the left side of the neck. Both the neck and abdomen should be draped in the sterile field (**Fig. 38-1**). The abdomen is entered through an upper midline incision and explored. The xiphoid process should be excised, a simple maneuver that greatly enhances exposure of the hiatus and gastroesophageal junction. The stomach must be completely mobilized so that it may be brought up to the neck based only on the right gastroepiploic artery.

The mobilization is begun by dividing the short gastric vessels so that this most difficult part of the gastric mobilization is completed first (**Fig. 38-2**). To bring the spleen up into a more favorable position, the left hand is placed laterally and posteriorly to the spleen and the spleen is lifted anteriorly and medially while laparotomy packs, rolled in thirds, are inserted posterior to the splenic hilum. Usually at least three of these packs are required to elevate the spleen enough to facilitate division of the short gastric vessels. Without these packs one is working deep within the abdomen, which in some patients is quite difficult and dangerous. The short gastric vessels are identified by incising the peritoneum between the greater curvature of the stomach and the spleen and individually identifying the vessels. With a right-angle clamp each vessel is encircled and tied in continuity, then divided. Four to five of these vessels should be identified. Once these are divided, the greater curvature is freed off the spleen and the packs behind the spleen are removed, allowing the spleen to return to its normal location. If the splenic capsule is torn, hemostasis should be achieved using electrocautery aided by hemostatic agents (Avitene or Surgicel) and packing. Rarely should it be necessary to perform a splenectomy unless there is a major laceration deep within the spleen or an injury to the hilum.

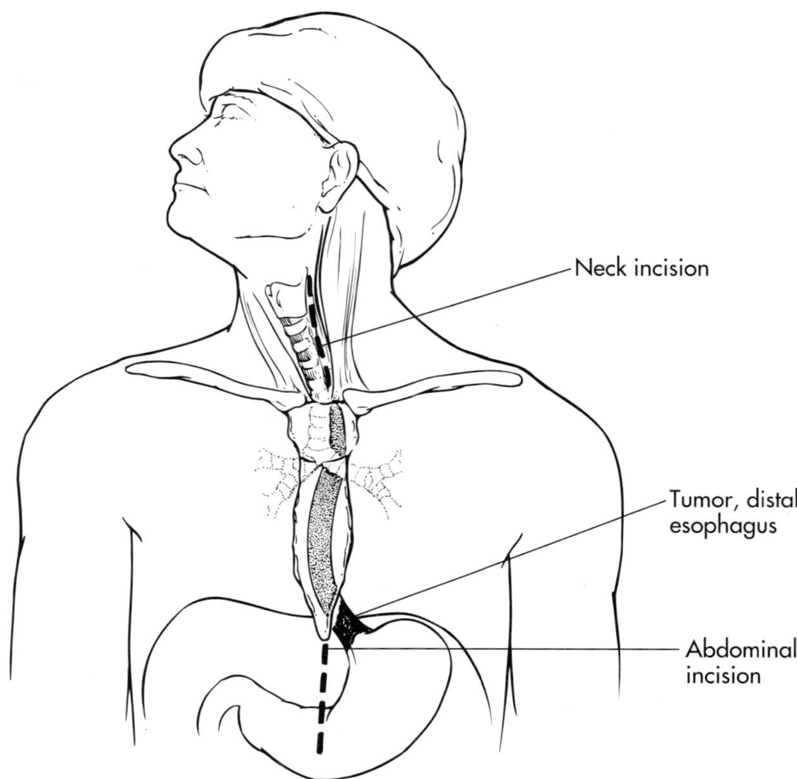

FIGURE 38-1

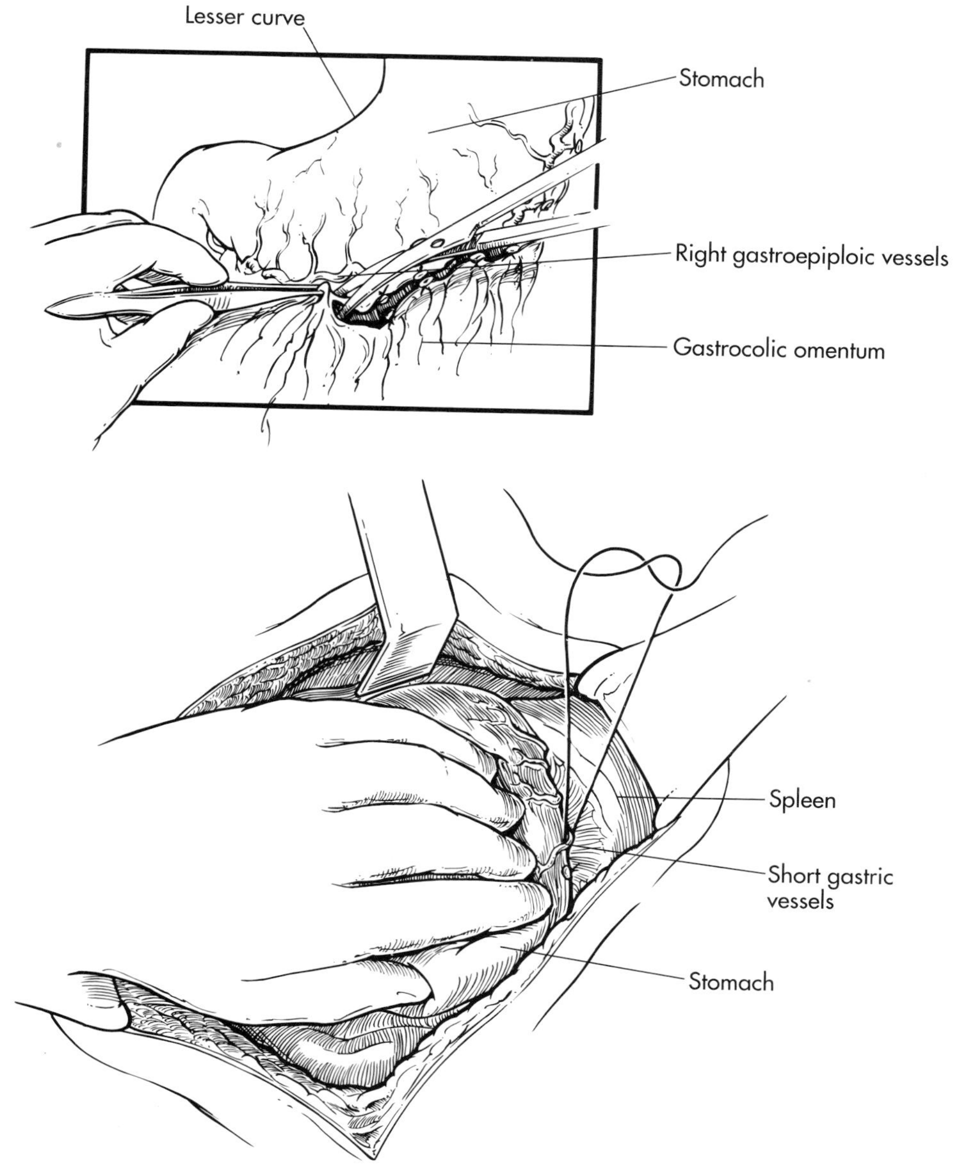

FIGURE 38-2

With the greater curvature of the stomach having been mobilized off the spleen, the lesser sac has been entered and it is now easy to divide the gastrocolic omentum (**Fig. 38-2, *inset***). Conversely, the gastric mobilization may be started by entering the lesser sac through the gastrocolic omentum and working up toward the spleen and back toward the pylorus. Great care must be taken to avoid the pedicle of the right gastroepiploic artery that runs along the greater curve. The pedicle is identified by both palpation and visualization. The gastrocolic omentum is divided by placing a series of clamps, dividing and ligating. Alternatively, a stapler that ligates and divides may also be used (LDS Stapler, US Surgical, Norwalk, Conn.). Care must be taken to avoid the transverse mesocolon, but there is a nice fusion plane that is readily identified between the omentum and the mesocolon. The omentum is divided back to the level of the pylorus, where the origin of the right gastroepiploic artery from the gastroduodenal artery is visualized.

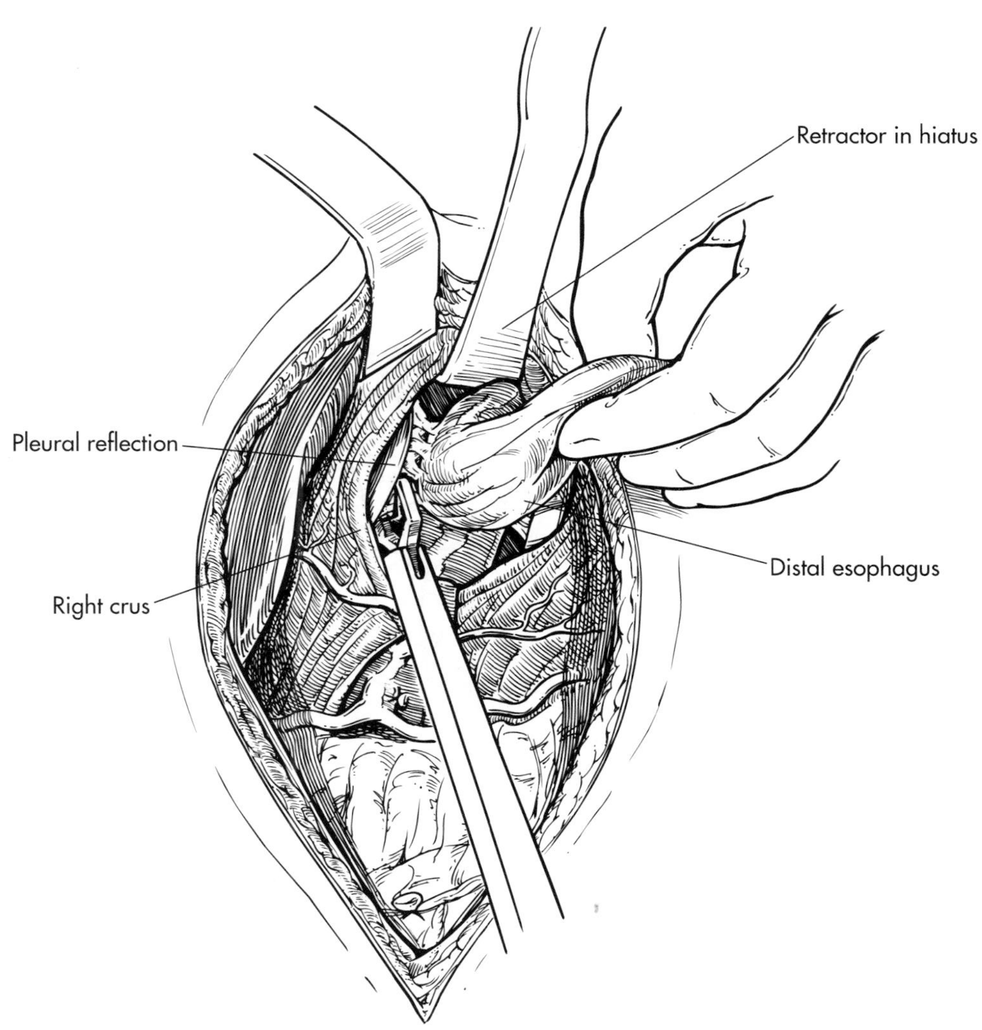
Retractor in hiatus
Pleural reflection
Distal esophagus
Right crus

FIGURE 38-5

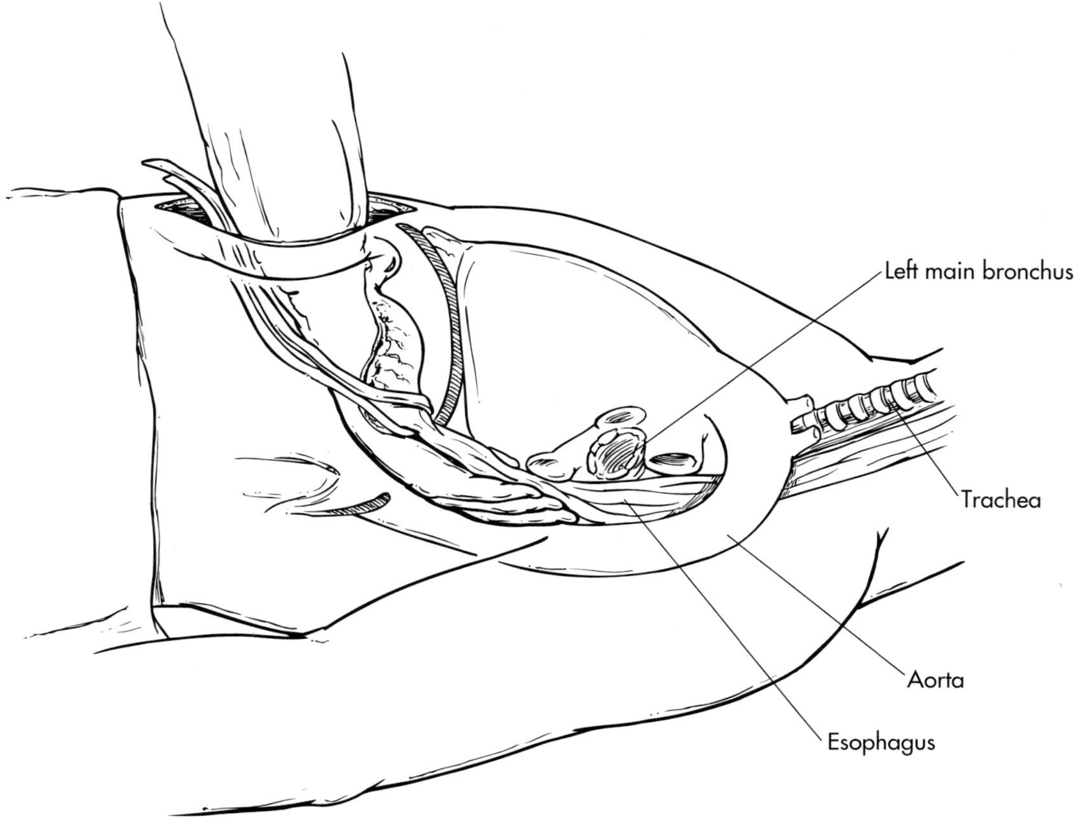

FIGURE 38-6

dissection should stay close to the wall of the esophagus to avoid injury to these adjacent structures. The major extent of the dissection is done from below, as described, and should be completed before dividing the lesser curve of the stomach since the traction achievable is greater with the esophagus and stomach intact.

Either a pyloromyotomy or pyloroplasty is performed to aid the drainage of the vagotomized stomach. Some surgeons argue against this practice, but it takes only one patient whose stomach does not empty to be convinced otherwise. The pyloromyotomy is performed by incising across the pylorus with approximately one third of the cut on the duodenal side and the rest on the gastric side. The duodenal mucosa is extremely thin and is easily entered if great care is not taken. The pyloric muscle band is easily seen and incised. A hemostat is placed within the line of excision and forcibly spread to tear the muscle band. Once the muscle band is penetrated, the mucosa is visualized and the myotomy is complete. The completeness is confirmed by placing the thumb and forefinger through the ring. If mucosa is entered inadvertently, the myotomy is converted to a pyloroplasty. The duodenum is fully mobilized by performing a Kocher maneuver, which allows the pylorus to come up to the level of the hiatus when the gastric remnant is transposed to the neck.

On the lesser curvature at the incisura, an area is cleared of omentum so that a linear stapler may be placed (**Fig. 38-7**). We use an 80-mm linear stapler with a 4.8-mm cartridge to remove the lesser curvature of the stomach. The line of division heads toward the apex of the greater curvature. If more length is necessary, it may be obtained by dividing more of the gastric remnant and narrowing the "tube." The staple line is begun at the incisura on the lesser curve and heads toward the greater curve instead of vice versa, since this maneuver seems to provide a small amount of additional length as it tends to slightly "straighten" the greater curve. Usually this division requires two firings of the stapler,

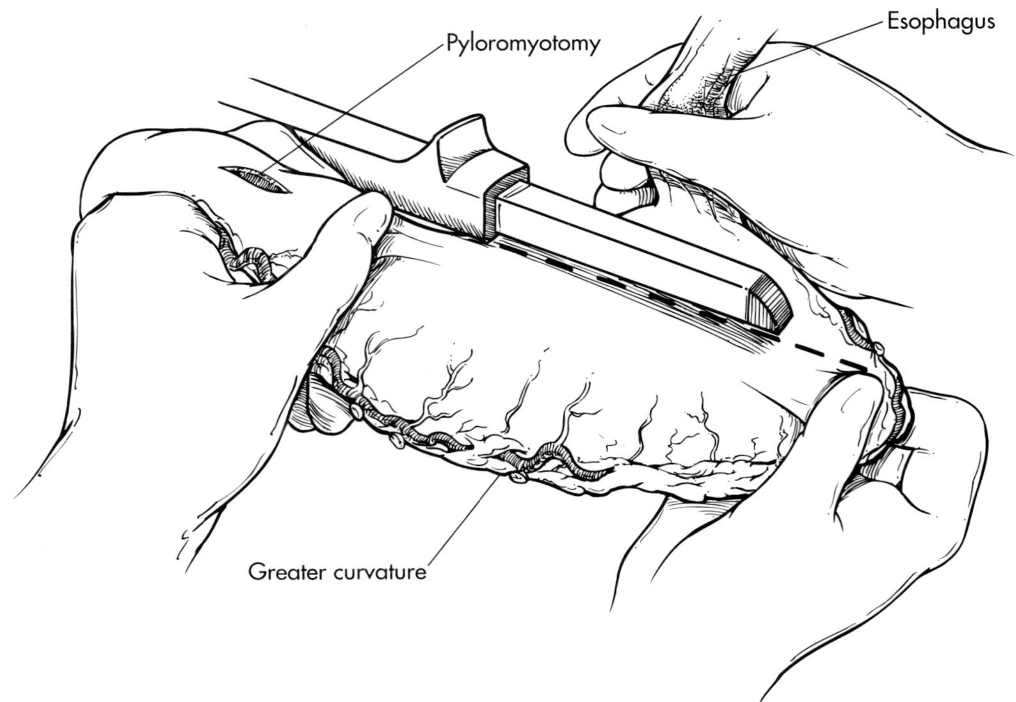
Pyloromyotomy
Esophagus
Greater curvature

FIGURE 38-7

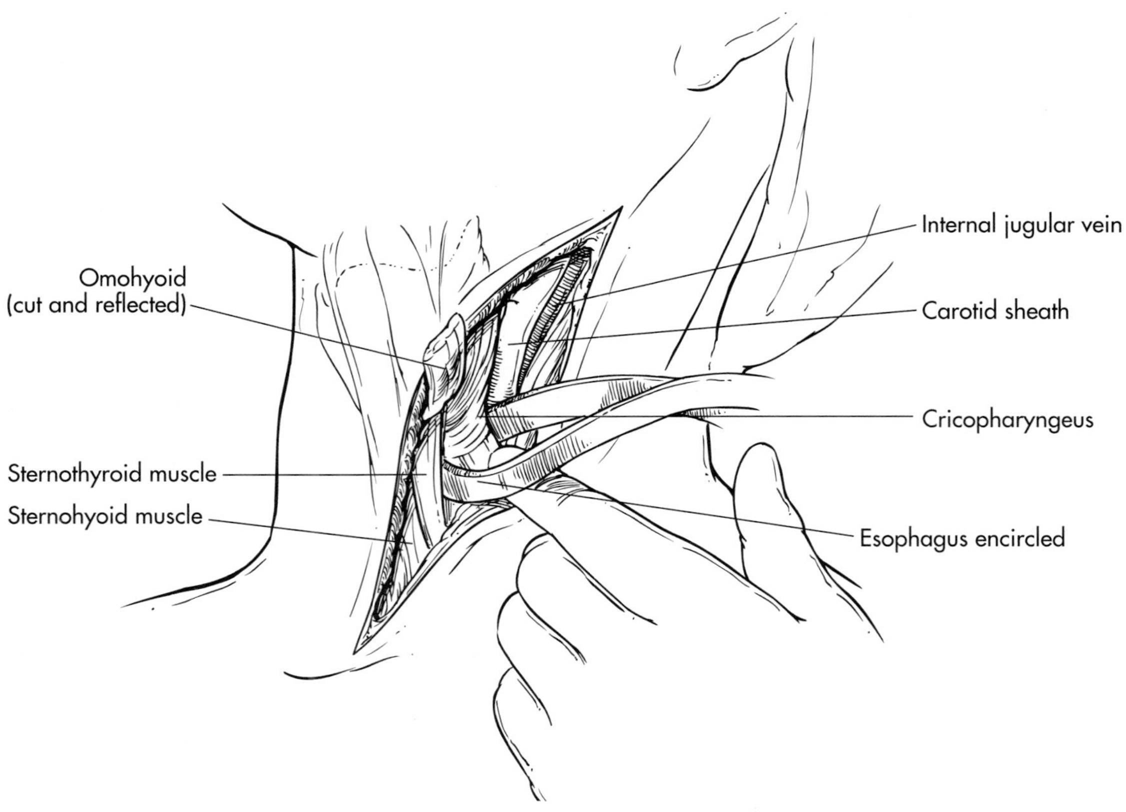
Omohyoid
(cut and reflected)
Internal jugular vein
Carotid sheath
Cricopharyngeus
Sternothyroid muscle
Sternohyoid muscle
Esophagus encircled

FIGURE 38-8

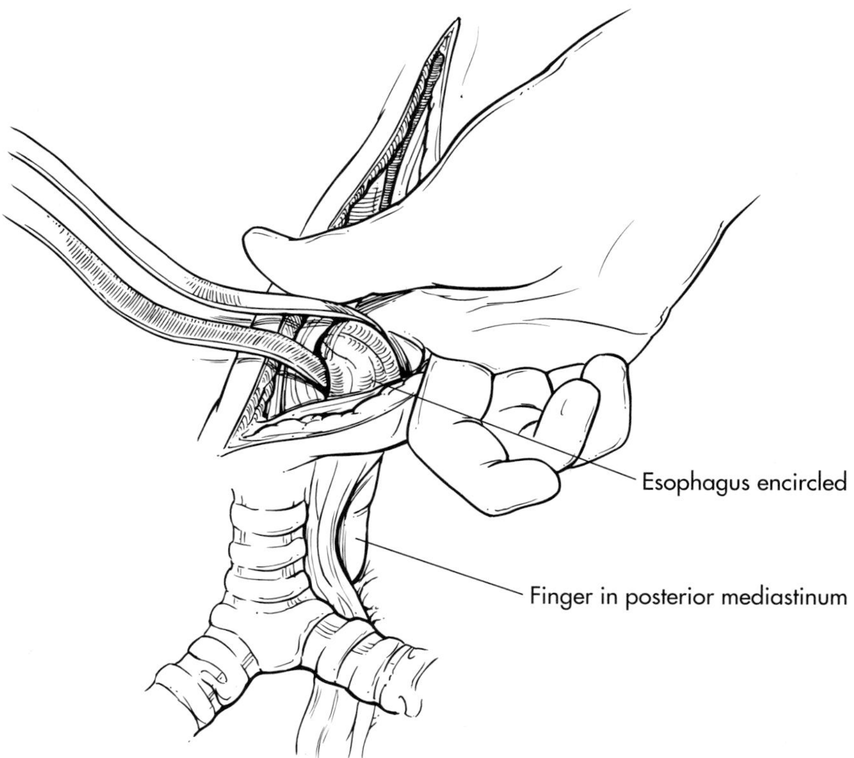

FIGURE 38-9

and I oversew the staple line with a continuous suture placed as seromuscular bites on each side of the staple line so as to cover it.

At this point attention is turned to the cervical portion of the procedure. A skin incision is made at the anterior border of the left sternocleidomastoid muscle, and the dissection is continued through the platysma. Dissection proceeds along the anterior border of the sternocleidomastoid medial to the carotid sheath down to the prevertebral fascia. The omohyoid muscle should be divided to enhance the exposure. The trachea is retracted with a finger toward the right, and the esophagus is encircled distal to the cricopharyngeus by carefully dissecting in the tracheoesophageal groove. Great care must be taken to avoid injury to the recurrent laryngeal nerve at this location. The dissection should stay on the wall of the esophagus, and a peanut sponge on a hemostat is used to dissect between the trachea and the esophagus in order to enter the plane to separate these structures. This dissection continues until the prevertebral fascia is seen on the opposite side of the esophagus. An angled clamp is used to pass a Penrose drain, to be used for traction, around the cervical esophagus (**Fig. 38-8**). Using a finger to dissect along the wall of the esophagus and pulling upward with the Penrose drain facilitates easy dissection of the proximal esophagus down to the level of the carina (**Fig. 38-9**). Combined dissection from above and below on all aspects of the esophagus allows the dissection to be completed (**Fig. 38-10**). Once completely free, the entire specimen is brought up through the mediastinum into the neck. An umbilical tape is attached to the distal esophagus before the specimen is pulled into the neck, and this is used to aid in bringing the gastric remnant into the neck.

To ensure adequate length of the gastric remnant, an estimation may be obtained by placing the gastric remnant on the chest, which is a significantly greater length than required to get to the neck via the posterior mediastinum (**Fig. 38-11**). If mobilized completely, the gastric remnant always reaches to the neck without tension. The pyloromyotomy should be at the level of the diaphragmatic hiatus. If there is any concern, one should check to make sure that complete mobilization has been obtained and then, perhaps, take off some more of the lesser curve, which usually produces some

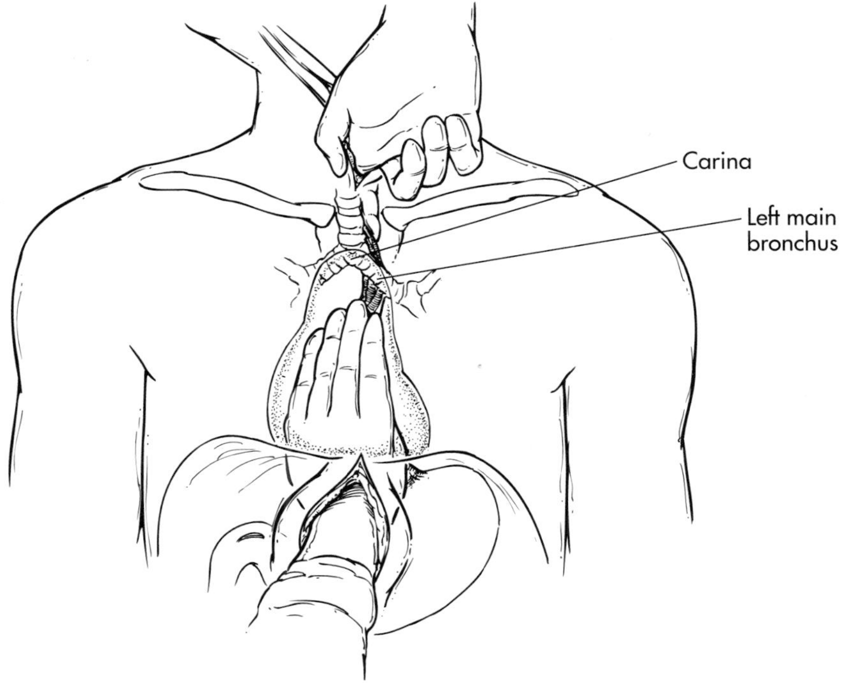

FIGURE 38-10

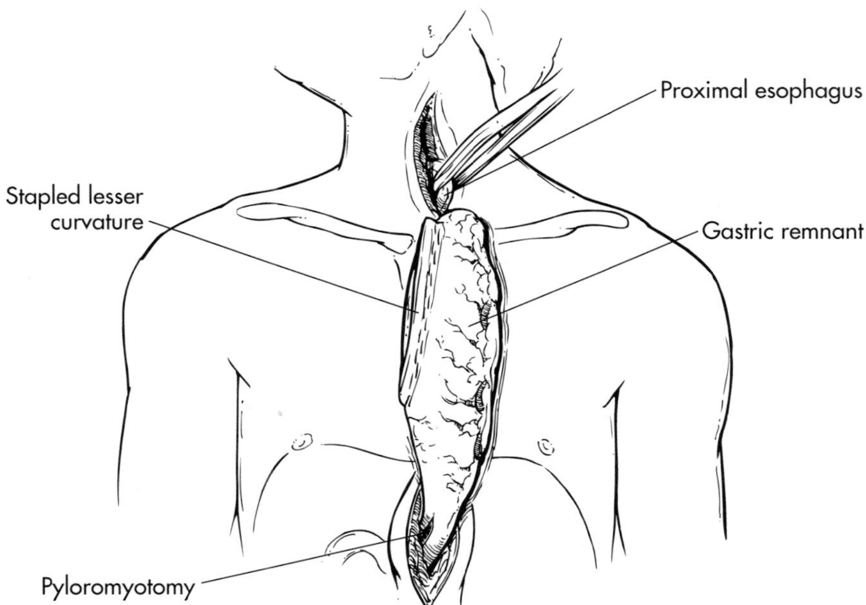

FIGURE 38-11

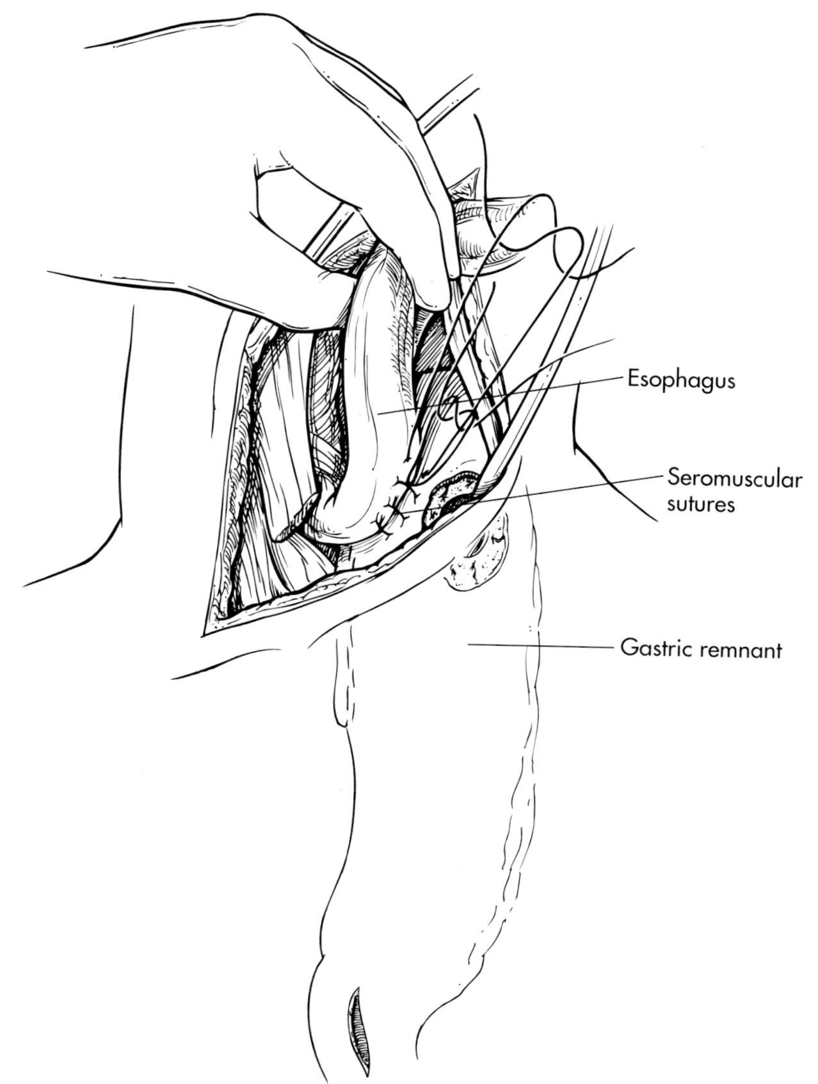

FIGURE 38-12

additional length. The gastric remnant is then brought through the posterior mediastinum up to the neck. This is done by placing the remnant into a plastic camera bag. The bag comes folded upon itself and expands to full length when pulled. The stomach is grasped with a Babcock clamp placed through the distal opening of the bag, and the stomach is drawn up into the bag. The umbilical tape previously passed through the posterior mediastinum is tied to the tip of the bag, not the stomach. Friction created between the dry surface of the stomach and the bag allows the stomach to be pulled up into the neck as the bag unfolds. This allows the gastric remnant to smoothly come through the mediastinum without the anterior or posterior wall "catching" and thus is fully extended. This results in more than enough length of stomach in the neck.

The gastric remnant is fixed in the neck by several sutures placed between it and the prevertebral fascia. I prefer to construct a hand-sewn anastomosis of either one or two layers, as described separately (**Fig. 38-12**). A nasogastric tube is placed through the anastomosis under direct vision before completion. The tube is positioned in the gastric remnant proximal to the pylorus. Once the anastomosis is completed, a suction drain is placed in the neck posterior to the anastomosis and directed inferiorly toward the posterior mediastinum and brought out through a separate stab wound. The

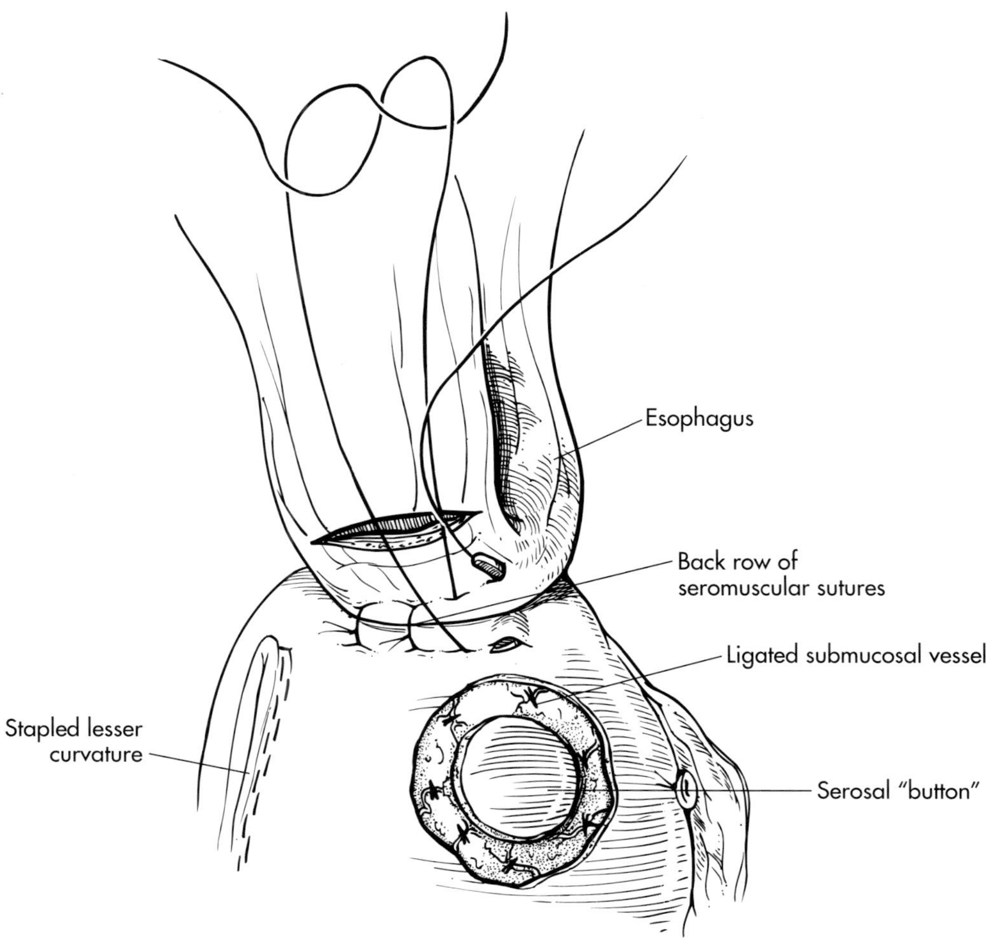
Esophagus
Back row of seromuscular sutures
Ligated submucosal vessel
Stapled lesser curvature
Serosal "button"

FIGURE 39-1

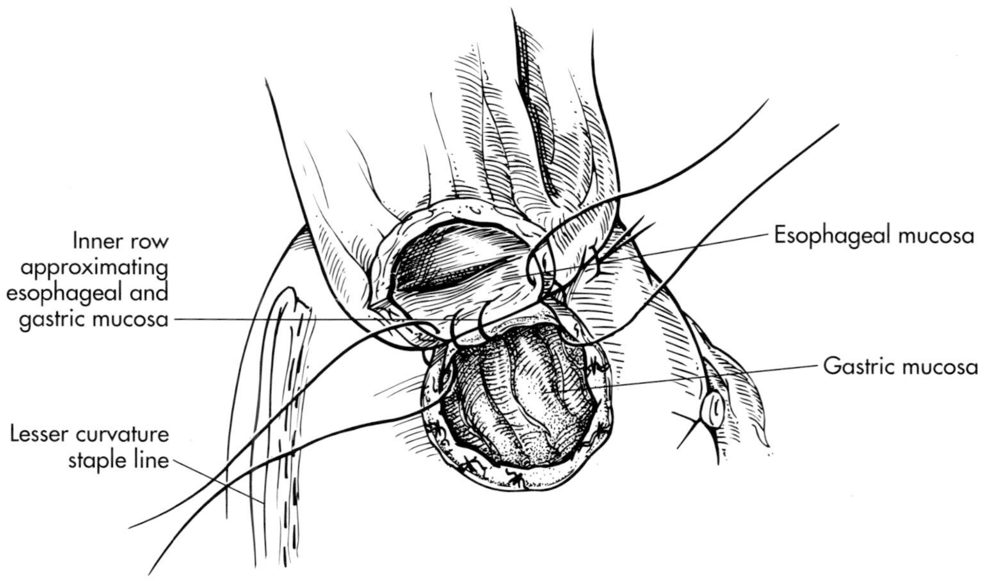
Inner row approximating esophageal and gastric mucosa
Esophageal mucosa
Gastric mucosa
Lesser curvature staple line

FIGURE 39-2

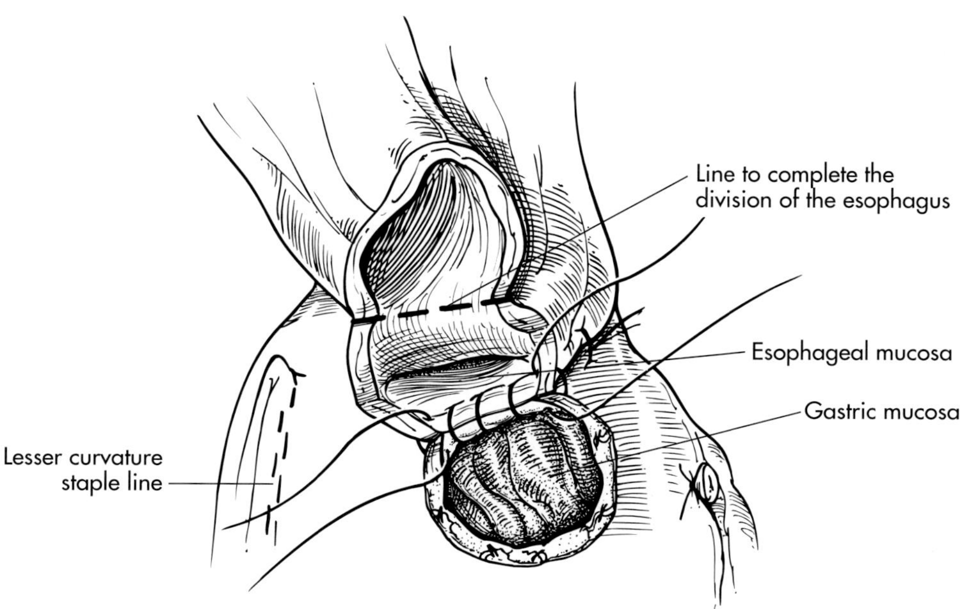
Line to complete the division of the esophagus
Esophageal mucosa
Gastric mucosa
Lesser curvature staple line

FIGURE 39-3

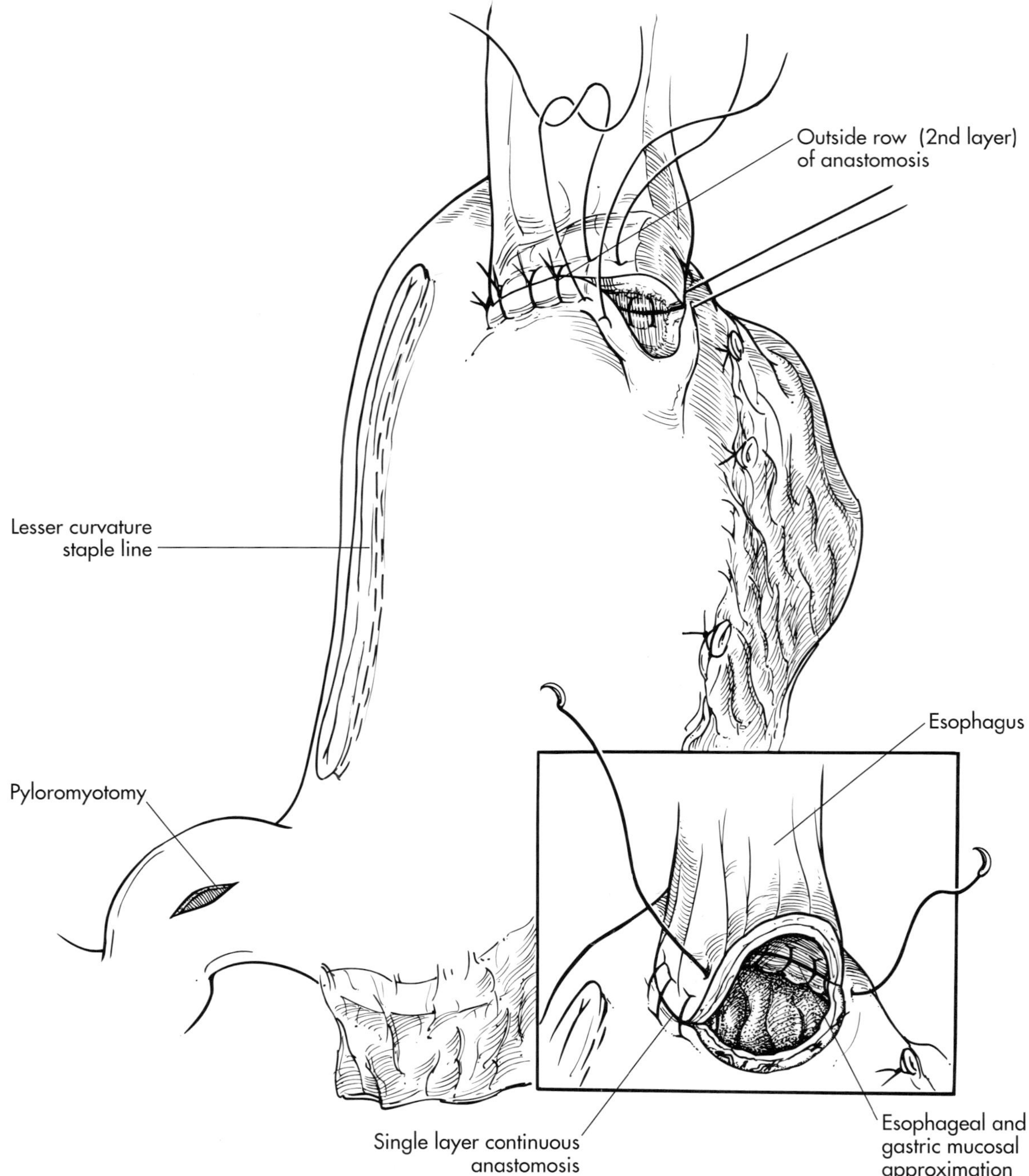

FIGURE 39-4

vision prior to the completion of this row of sutures. A few sutures are placed but not tied, and the anastomosis is completed with the placement of a Connell stitch (inside out, outside in on one side, then inside out, outside in on the other side). The last few sutures are tied after the Connell stitch. The anastomosis is completed by placing a second layer, which encompasses seromuscular bites of the gastric remnant and muscularis bites of the esophagus. The gastric side should be brought up to the esophagus, not vice versa. The anastomosis must not be under any tension at completion.

The anastomosis may also be constructed in one layer using a continuous suture, which is my current preference (**Fig. 39-4, *inset***). Again, the mucosa-to-mucosa approximation is the key to the anastomosis. The esophagus must be completely transected to begin this anastomosis, and either a double-armed stitch or two sutures are placed at the midpoint of the back row. The stitch is placed in an inverting fashion to bring the mucosal edges together, and one end, or one suture, is run toward each corner with each bite encompassing all layers on each side. Precise suture placement is the key. For this anastomosis a monofilament absorbable material is the preferred suture. Tension is maintained on the suture as the anastomosis is constructed. Purse-stringing is not a problem with an anastomosis constructed in this way since, once a few throws have been placed, the suture does not slide. Once the entire circumference is completed, the two ends of the two sutures are tied together, completing the anastomosis.

This anastomotic technique applies in all esophageal resections no matter the operative approach chosen or the location of the anastomosis.

Bibliography

Akiyama H: Esophageal anastomosis, *Arch Surg* 107:512–515, 1973.

Mathisen DJ, Grillo HC, Wilkins EW, et al: Transthoracic esophagectomy: a safe approach to carcinoma of the esophagus, *Ann Thorac Surg* 45:137–140, 1988.

Sweet RH: Carcinoma of the esophagus and cardiac end of the stomach: immediate and late results of treatment by resection and primary esophagogastric anastomosis, *JAMA* 135:485–491, 1947.

CHAPTER 40

Esophagectomy Via Laparotomy and Right Thoracotomy

Esophagectomy via laparotomy and right thoracotomy is the most versatile of all the approaches to esophagectomy, since it is useful for esophageal lesions in any location. The gastroesophageal junction is difficult to expose through the right side of the chest, but this area of the resection is well exposed at laparotomy. The disadvantage to this approach is the necessity to change the position of the patient during the operation, which increases the length of the procedure. Also, the necessity of opening two body cavities potentially subjects the patient to increased morbidity. This approach is particularly useful for midesophageal lesions in close proximity to the carina. As part of the preoperative evaluation patients with midesophageal lesions should undergo bronchoscopy to determine whether there is evidence of invasion of the airway of either the trachea or left main bronchus. Invasion of the airway precludes resection so this determination is an important part of the evaluation.

DESCRIPTION OF THE PROCEDURE

In most cases the patient is placed on the operating table in the supine position, and the abdominal portion of the operation is completed first. This involves complete mobilization of the stomach and dissection of the esophagus at the hiatus, as described in the section on transhiatal esophagectomy. A pyloromyotomy or pyloroplasty is done, and the duodenum is mobilized with a Kocher maneuver. The esophagus is mobilized at the hiatus and dissected as far up as possible into the chest. This dissection up into the chest is extremely important given the difficulty in accessing the hiatus provided by the right thoracotomy.

The gastric remnant is prepared before closing the abdomen. The lesser curve of the stomach is divided with several applications of a linear stapler, starting at the incisura and extending up to the apex of the stretched out stomach as described in the chapter on transhiatal esophagectomy. It is far easier to complete this division via the laparotomy than to try to do this in the chest. The staple line is oversewn with a continuous stitch taking seromuscular bites on each side of the staple line, which results in the staple line being covered. A feeding jejunostomy tube is placed, and the abdomen is closed.

The patient is then placed in the left lateral decubitus position after placement of a left endobronchial double-lumen tube for single-lung ventilation. A right posterolateral thoracotomy incision is made and the chest entered through the 6th intercostal space (**Fig. 40-1**). Entering the chest at a lower interspace makes the dissection of the proximal esophagus somewhat more difficult. Entry through the 5th intercostal space is acceptable as long as the distal esophagus has been well dissected from below. A vertical axillary muscle-sparing incision may also be used, and it results in excellent exposure of the posterior mediastinum. The pleura overlying the esophagus is incised, and the esophagus is dissected off the aorta and the trachea (**Fig. 40-2**). It is helpful to

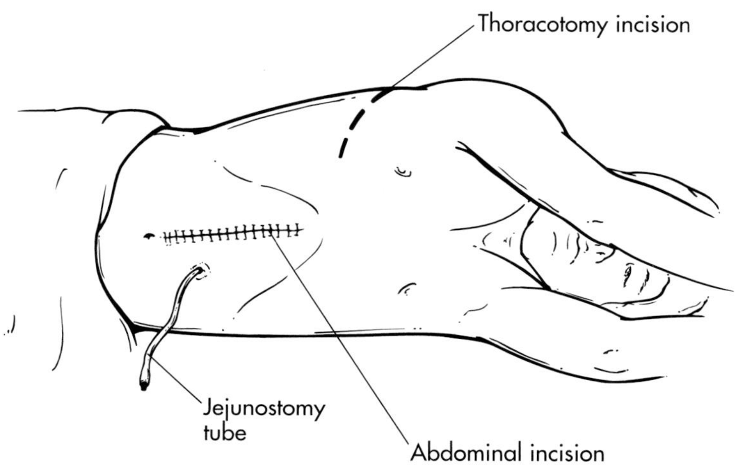

FIGURE 40-1

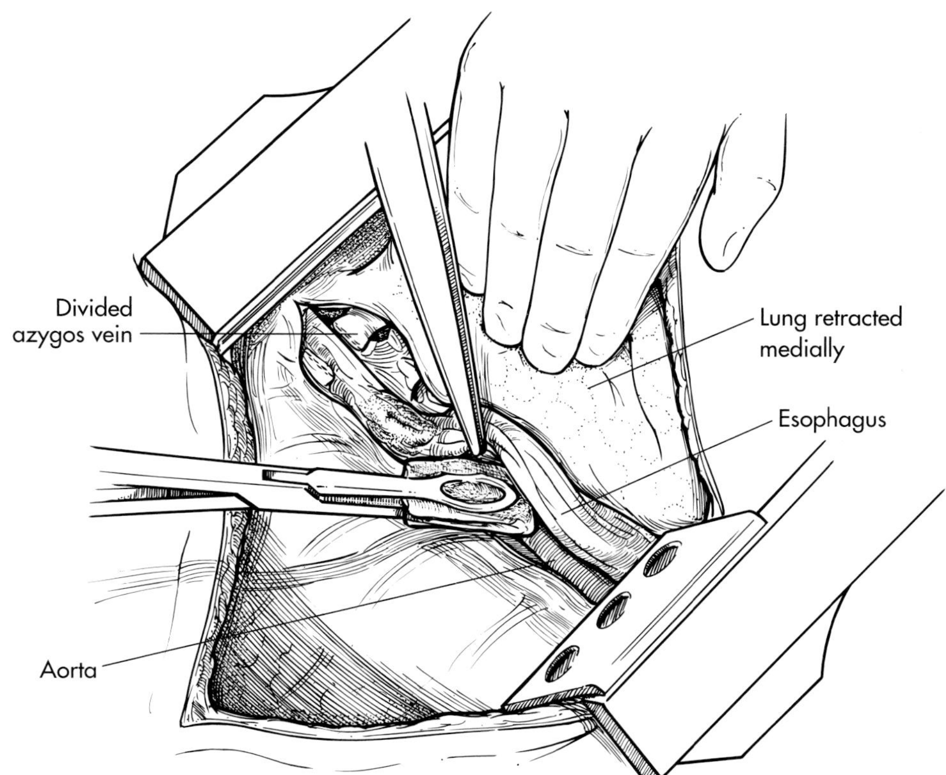

FIGURE 40-2

C H A P T E R 41

Esophagectomy Via Left Thoracotomy

Distal esophageal lesions, particularly lesions of the gastroesophageal junction, may be managed solely through a left thoracotomy with the abdominal portion performed either through the hiatus or, preferably, through a rent made in the hemidiaphragm. To some surgeons this approach is preferred for most esophageal lesions. Lesions of the midesophagus and even those at the level of the inferior pulmonary vein are difficult to manage through this approach because of the position of the aortic arch. The arch makes lesions at the level of the carina essentially inaccessible from the left side of the chest. Constructing an anastomosis just inferior to the aortic arch is difficult, especially from a 6th intercostal space incision, which is the preferred space for entering the chest. Thus I reserve this approach for select distal esophageal lesions, mainly gastroesophageal junction lesions, where the aortic arch does not interfere and the anastomosis can be constructed in a convenient location within the chest.

DESCRIPTION OF THE PROCEDURE

The patient is placed on the operating table in the right lateral decubitus position after placement of a left endobronchial double-lumen tube for single-lung ventilation. A posterolateral thoracotomy incision is made and the chest entered through the 6th or 7th intercostal space (**Fig. 41-1**). If necessary, the incision can be extended across the costal arch as a thoracoabdominal incision, with the

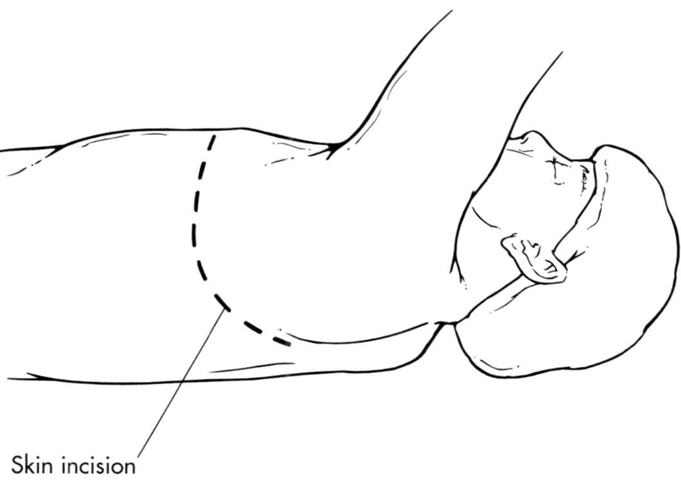

FIGURE 41-1

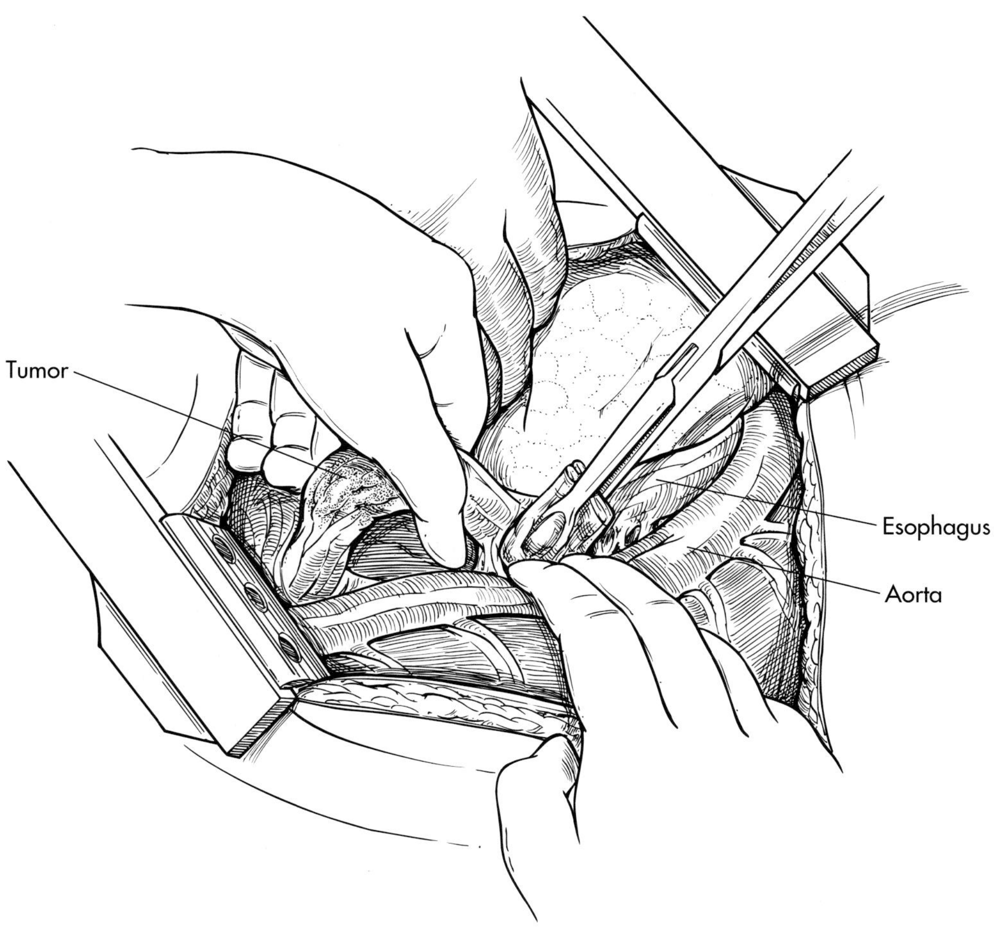

FIGURE 41-2

abdominal portion stopping lateral to the rectus muscle. The mediastinal pleura overlying the esophagus is incised and the esophagus mobilized (**Fig. 41-2**). It is best to begin this mobilization away from the tumor, because a Penrose drain placed around the esophagus away from the tumor can be used for traction to facilitate the esophageal dissection. I often begin this dissection by grasping the pericardium with a Kocher clamp, and with upward traction applied, I dissect pleura just at the pericardium, which quickly reveals the esophagus. For most gastroesophageal junction lesions the esophagus needs to be mobilized only as high as the aortic arch, though some surgeons are content to go only slightly above the level of the inferior pulmonary vein.

The diaphragm is incised in a circumferential fashion away from the central portion. At times the gastric mobilization may be completed through the hiatus, but I prefer to open the diaphragm because I think it offers better exposure (**Fig. 41-3**). The short gastric vessels are easily visualized, since one is basically looking down onto the stomach. These vessels are divided first, and the mobilization of the greater curvature proceeds from the cardia toward the antrum. This mobilization is performed as described in Chapter 38, detailing transhiatal esophagectomy. As the greater curvature is mobilized, the stomach can be delivered into the chest, and either a pyloromyotomy or pyloroplasty is performed (**Fig. 41-4**). The gastric remnant is fashioned in the usual way with several firings of the linear stapler from the incisura to the apex of the greater curvature. A one- or two-layer hand-sewn anastomosis is then constructed at an appropriate level (**Fig. 41-5**). At times another intercostal space (usually the fourth) may need to be opened in order to construct the anastomosis at the level of the aortic arch. If necessary, an anastomosis may be performed above the arch by dissecting circumferentially around the aortic

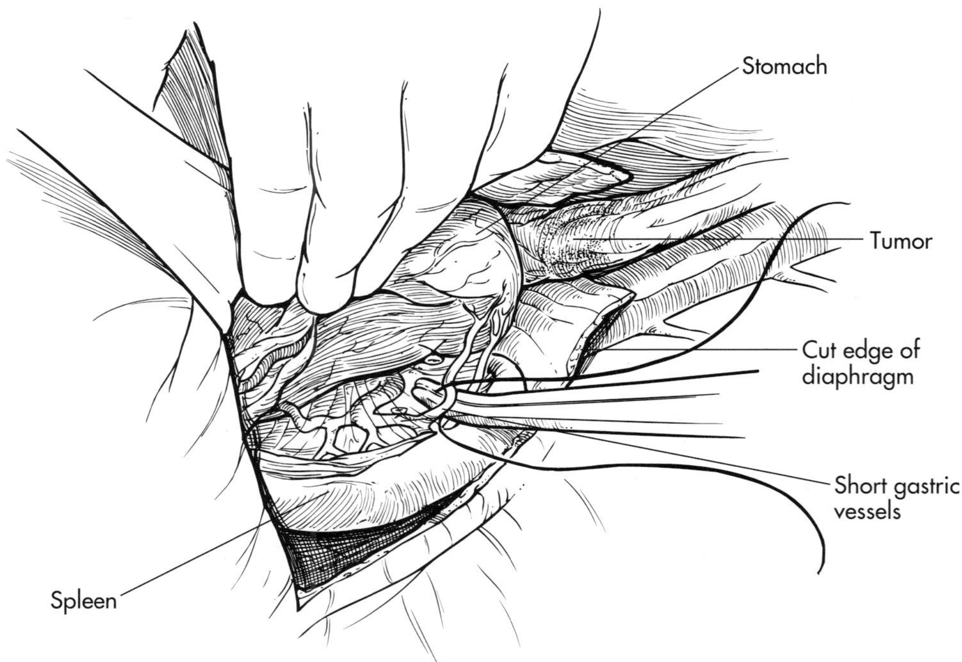

FIGURE 41-3

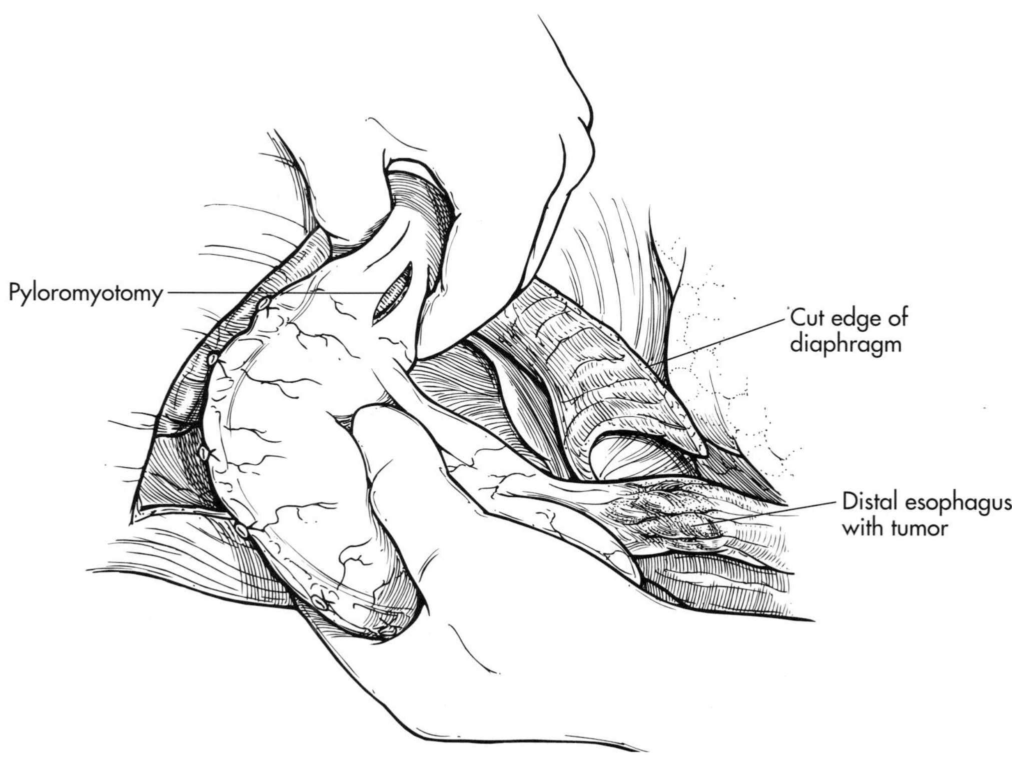

FIGURE 41-4

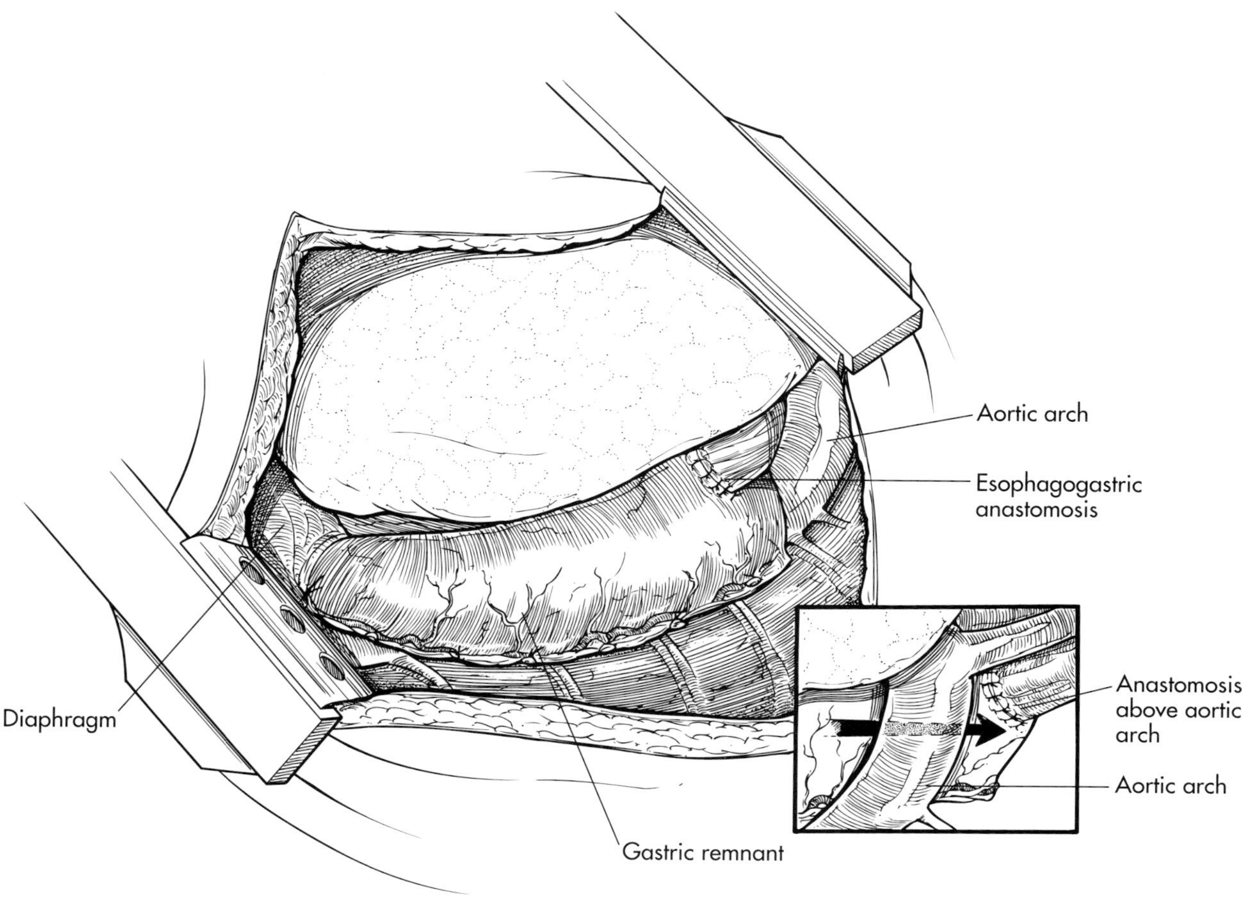

FIGURE 41-5

arch and bringing the gastric remnant through this posterior tunnel (**Fig. 41-5, *inset***). When dissecting deep to the aortic arch, metal clips should be used liberally and one should be aware that the thoracic duct may be located in close proximity. An anastomosis at this level almost always mandates opening an additional higher intercostal space, as mentioned above.

If esophagectomy is being performed for an adenocarcinoma arising in a columnar-lined esophagus (Barrett's esophagus), it is necessary to resect all of the esophagus that contains this abnormal mucosa that has already undergone malignant change in at least one location. This may require total esophagectomy with an anastomosis in the neck. The patient will have to be moved to the supine position in order to complete the neck dissection and anastomosis. This, of course, is time-consuming, and in these cases transhiatal esophagectomy may be the better procedure. Again, this underscores the importance of the esophageal surgeon being well versed in all approaches to resection of this difficult organ and to have thought carefully about the approach before beginning the procedure.

A feeding jejunostomy tube is placed, and the rent in the diaphragm is repaired with a continuous stitch of heavy monofilament suture. Two chest tubes are placed, and the intercostal space is reapproximated with paracostal sutures. If a second intercostal space has been opened, it is necessary to place paracostal sutures in that location as well. The rest of the closure is as per the routine for thoracotomy.

Bibliography

Page RD, Khalil JF, Whyte RI, et al: Esophagogastrectomy via left thoracophrenotomy, *Ann Thorac Surg* 49:763, 1990.

Wilkins EW Jr: Left thoracoabdominal approaches. In Pearson FG, Deslauriers J, Ginsberg RJ, et al, eds: *Esophageal surgery*, New York, 1995, Churchill Livingstone.

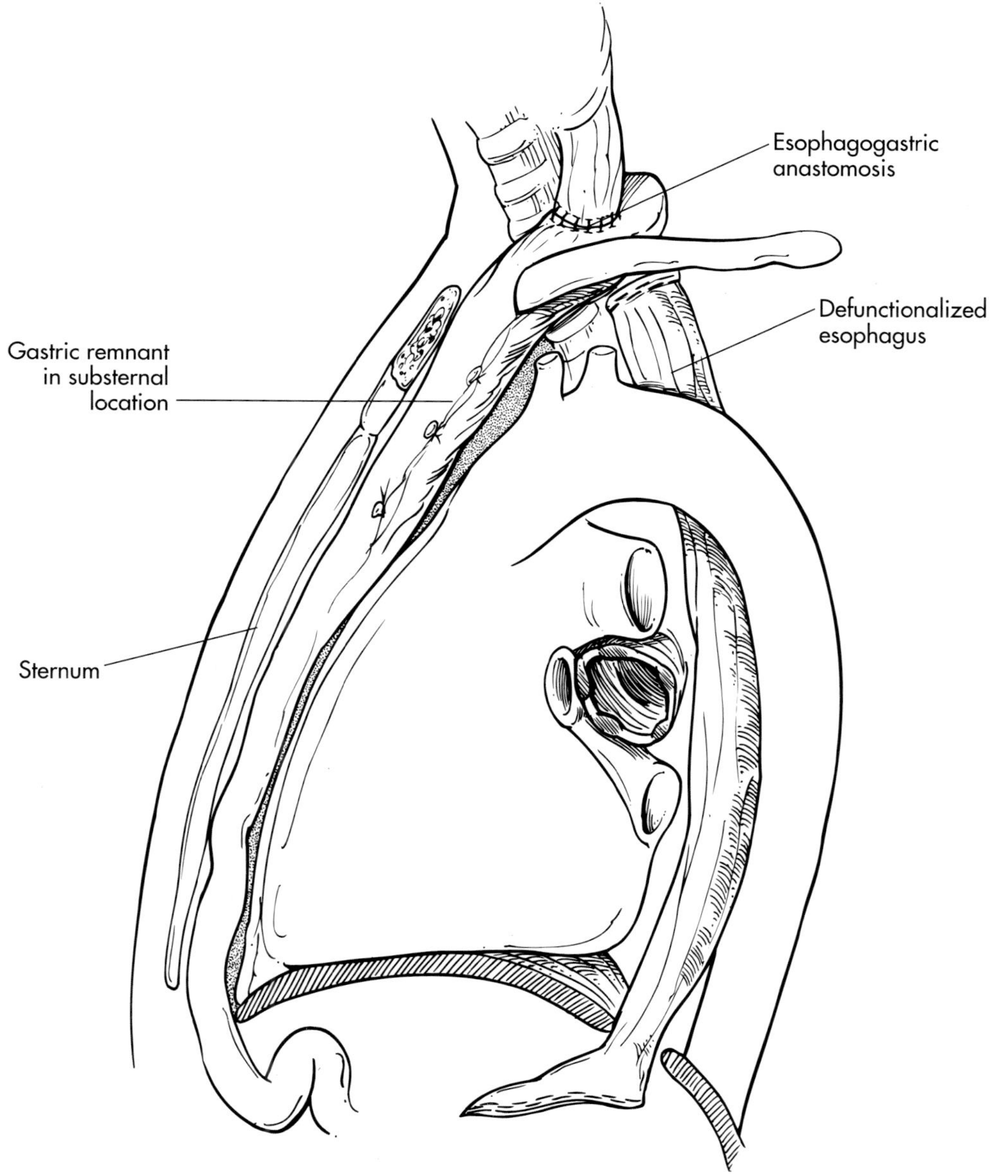

FIGURE 42-4

Before completion of the anastomosis, a nasogastric tube is inserted and positioned just proximal to the pylorus. A suction drain is left in the neck.

Substernal gastric bypass is associated with a high incidence of morbidity, mainly because of the patients who are candidates for the procedure. Great care should be taken in selecting patients for this procedure. For the right patient it provides excellent palliation, a benefit well worth the risk of the procedure.

Bibliography

Little AG and Kirgan D: Bypass and intubation. In Pearson FG, Deslauriers J, Ginsberg RJ, et al, eds: *Esophageal surgery*, New York, 1995, Churchill Livingstone.

Mannell A, Becker P, and Nissenbaum M: Bypass surgery for unresectable oesophageal cancer: early and late results in 124 cases, *Br J Surg* 75:283, 1988.

Robinson J, Isu S, Everett M, et al: Substernal gastric bypass for palliation of esophageal carcinoma: rationale and technique, *Surgery* 97:305, 1981.

INDEX

NOTE—Page numbers in **boldface** indicate illustrations.